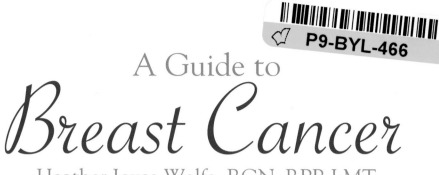
A Guide to
Breast Cancer

Heather Joyce Wolfe, RGN, RPP, LMT

A Whole Body A–Z
for Prevention and Healing

A Conventional and Alternative Approach

First Edition October 2010

First published in 2010 by Back to Source Books
www.backtosource.com

Text by Heather Joyce Wolfe
Photographs by Jess Walsh

Layout and design by Carolyn Connors, Gloucester, MA USA

Printed in Ireland by KPS Colour Print, Knock, Co. Mayo. Ireland

Text copyright © 2010 by H. J. Wolfe
Photographs copyright © 2010 by Jess Walsh

ISBN# 978-0-9567243-0-4

FOR MY CHILDREN,
ROSS AND ANNA KRACHEY

Preface

Searching for Silver Linings and the Soul...

Dear Reader,

Thank you for picking up this book. It is my wish that there will be at least one item in it that will bring you better health, more joy, peace and true connection with your Self and your Source of Life, whatever you wish to call this – Great Spirit, God, Allah, Holy Spirit or Love.

I do not pretend to know or understand everything on the subject of cancer, and neither do I know anyone who does. I respect those who have done their homework. I am wary of the influence of drug companies who stand to make millions on various synthetic medications, valid as some of them may be. Studies published are generally done on the synthetics, rather than natural substances, so there is an imbalance in this arena. In this book I hope to make the slate a little cleaner so that people know that there is more choice available, should they seek it.

The causes and cures for cancer are known by quite a number of people, and have been known for some time. There needs to be different strokes for different folks, and life manifests at varied vibrations and levels of consciousness. Each of us has different requirements for our learning experiences at different times.

Illness, pain and death can be transformative and we still seem to need them for our growth. Otherwise, at this stage of our evolution, I think we may become complacent. Hard times challenge us to change and remind us to ask for Grace, Mercy and God, whoever and whatever that is for any one of us. Perhaps as we learn more about each of these and pay more attention, let go of old patterns, listen to ourselves and Mother Earth, we will not need illness and all it brings with it.

Since the present epidemic of breast cancer is affecting so many women, (and some men) and potentially many more, it seems that we have an opportunity and responsibility to find a way through this shocking dilemma in which we find ourselves, one woman at a time, with honesty, courage, compassion and vulnerability.

For now, if we accept our plight as well as fight it, and are willing to face our shadow as individuals, a race and a planet, and can learn to trust the process and open our minds to new possibilities everywhere, we may be able to create bodies that are immune to disease.

Many cultures, notably the Mayans, say that we are coming to the end of a Dark Age in December 2012, and beginning a new more enlightened one. That gives us very little time to wrap up the darkness! No wonder the pace is rather fast, and shadows are coming to the light for healing.

It is time to take care of each other, and for each of us to share our gifts in a way that brings us Love, Joy and Peace.

My journey with cancer and recovery has been over three years long now, with a lot of change and learning in the process. I procrastinated. I went into overwhelm and didn't pay attention to my body, even though it was crying out for attention. I did give it quite a fair amount, but not enough for my particular needs. I created a blatant split in myself – where one part of me knew that I wasn't as well as I could be, and another just kept going due to subconscious fear and old habitual patterning, which could be called addiction. I finally took the time to find out what was going on, and to face the fact that I had a small lump in my left breast, which upon investigation showed malignancy. I had had trouble with a cyst here in previous years.

Cancer can kill, so a sentence of death is possible with the diagnosis. I didn't want to die, for many reasons, though a part of me was a little ambivalent about living. I had the right ingredients for my wake up call – despair, resentment, resistance and conflict, mostly within myself, though well reflected outside. These took their toll over time, with some other added ingredients. I explored them to the nth degree, recognising my own uniqueness. I am a strong woman in many ways, with a very delicate energy system, and my own weaknesses – all needing consideration.

In the medical profession I found skilled loving care and support. My surgeon was tops, and never allowed his eyelids to bat as I shared that I had actually known that I was cancer positive from the medical clairvoyant reading I had the previous day! He educated me with all the options and listened to mine. I didn't know a definite path, though I was aware of options that could possibly do the job, (no guarantees) were I willing and able. Being faced with decisions for oneself is vastly different than for someone else. I am not someone else.

When the small lump was removed from my breast, the sentinel lymph node from under my left arm was also removed and found to contain a few cancerous cells.

I did know, through clairvoyance, that there were no more cancer cells in the remaining (axilliary) lymph nodes under my arm. I was told that Orthodox Medicine had no way of examining the nodes at that time, other than removing them, and statistics showed that I had a 14% chance of having more abnormal cells. I experienced some confusion, conflict and fear that would not allow me to cancel my second surgery. I opted for this. Two weeks later I was informed that no further cancer cells were found.

I chose to spend much time alone in recovery, doing what I had been yearning to do – spending time in solitude and prayer, with my favourite music, in my room overlooking the ocean, where I had seen many people for their healing. Now it was my turn. I relished this time, despite the considerable pain of getting my range of motion back after removal of my lymph nodes.

If I had not opted to have this second operation (considered major surgery) I probably would not have had the impetus to write this book, so there was a silver lining – for many I hope, and certainly myself, still being revealed.

Whether I hadn't the guts to say no to that second surgery, or my gut was saying yes, was a question for me. I honoured the flow of energy that was happening, for whatever reason.

I surrendered.

My gut was absolutely sure that it did not want chemotherapy or radiation as suggested. I did not feel that I would survive it. I didn't feel that my immune system was strong enough, and physically I felt too weak. I needed more time to recuperate before making that kind of decision.

I used every bit of knowledge that I possessed, both from the wisdom of my nursing background, and much that I had learned and practiced in the field of alternative healing to guide my own path to recovery. My love of music and sound served me well, along with meditation and the power of mind over matter in the form of guided meditation and self hypnosis. I found a nutritionist who tested me with kinesiology for my nutrition and supplements. I received gentle hands on healing. I let go of much that had been depleting my energy field and causing geopathic stress, so that I could restore my health and come into balance. I sought help psychologically, as well as coaching, to move forward in my life. I directed specific colours into my energy field and became aware of the importance of the vibration of each one for my healing.

I studied books on cancer, while trying to keep a positive attitude and release any fear – not an easy task. I consulted several clairvoyants who told me what they saw, especially those who knew how to see the vibration of cancer, and/or cancer cells, and listened to their suggestions for improving my situation, while keeping tabs on myself with my doctor through blood tests, breast examination and mammograms, and valued the support I got here. I also discover the AMAS blood test for cancer cells (available only in the USA) and found that it was within normal limits, which was very reassuring.

I knew that my immune system was vastly influenced by my state of mind, and was aware of when I needed help with this, and asked for it. My own Biofeedback device was helpful in showing me truth, and my detox footbath helped keep my system clean with a more alkaline pH. I had paid attention to the water I drank for many years, but now I learned more about this and it became all-important. The air I breathed, and didn't breathe, was a barometer for feeling good, or not.

I rarely ate (eat) any food that was not organic, and I learned more deeply the importance of this. Chopping and juicing vegetables (not fruit, except for the odd apple) became a wonderful daily ritual. I added more sprouts of various kinds as a scrumptious meal in themselves!

I used plants in the form of essential oils and flower remedies, as well as herbal tinctures. Homeopathic remedies played an important role at certain stages in my journey, though I now know that they work optimally in a properly hydrated body, and this was not always my case.

I noticed how difficult it is to live in a healthy environment in our current world compared to life during my childhood, though not impossible – just requiring more mindfulness and consciousness, which can become good practice for enlightenment – another silver lining!

Fear was a regular visitor because of the stress that I knew I was still enduring, and the knowledge that this was conducive to the growth of cancer cells, and to an acid system, also unfavourable. If I had a fight it was to keep this stress under control. I used my own resources, but most valuable were those of others in the alternative healing arts, which I absolutely knew made all the difference. The downside to this is that there was a financial drain, which can be incredibly stressful, and so the balance was always precarious. However there are many things one can do which do not cost anything, or cost very little, except your time and commitment, which can be a huge commitment in itself. I was grateful for some Government agencies, as well as charitable organizations, for support in this way.

One of the greatest assets of living in our time, in western culture anyway, is the freedom of choice that we have, though it can also be confusing. We have the potential for clarity if we have the knowledge of what is available, and so I hope that the information contained in these pages will give you that in a clear, efficient and concise way on the much talked about subject of breast cancer – that it will save some time and anxiety, and allow conscious choices to be made.

My sense is that breast cancer is a wake up call for women all over the world to come back to what we know deep down inside. This is unique for each one of us, and also has a common denominator which connects us all. Perhaps we can turn this disease around so that we will connect through prevention rather than illness. That would be my hope for the not very distant future. We are the ones who can choose.

Can we learn what we need to learn without experiencing breast cancer? Perhaps enough of us have done this journey of self discovery now to allow this to happen.

I have come to know that cancer has the ability to bring us to our Soul's potential, if we allow it. This requires commitment, attention, and willingness to face ourselves and our subconscious, sometimes with more speed than we would otherwise have mustered. With these three qualities come all the support that is needed. This is the Law of Energy and Attraction.

All systems of healing and medicine have miracles to offer, as well as excellent skill and care. As minds and hearts open, fear is lessened by education and experience. Gradually we will come together to find the best, simplest and most compassionate way, as well as the most economical, to provide preventive, corrective and palliative health care for all.

Experience becomes wisdom. May it be so….

Almost every day I meet people who tell me they know someone who died of breast cancer, or who has just been diagnosed, or is undergoing treatment. This always spurs me on to find more information primarily on the cause of this disease. Despite all the efforts spent in researching and treating breast cancer worldwide, why is it we still have 1.2 million deaths annually, and many more suffering?

There is learning in all of it, and perhaps we can find a different, more joyful way, if we could commit to that. It is called PREVENTION. This is not about early detection, which is certainly a step in the right direction, and has given life to many, including me. How would it be if we didn't need that as much, or if less disease were detected? It would be more economical for sure, and perhaps it is economics that will get us there in the end. Each individual must ask her/himself this question. It is a Soul question, and an act of Self Love. However, we have many ways to sabotage ourselves, and many veils covering our eyes and ears, most of which we are unaware. This is the adventure – going deep down inside ourselves until we find the jewel in there that shines so brightly that no disease can reside in this vibration.

There is quite a lot to read between these covers for all levels of your Being, and it can take some time to read it all – time that you may not have in this moment, so if you feel inclined please open to a page or a letter of the alphabet (try the contents?) and see what it has to say to you. I always liked games, and cards surrounded me when growing up, one way or another, and this is my game for you!

Remember to keep looking for those Silver Linings….and to keep smiling, keep moving, keep alkaline and keep hydrated!

Love and Blessings
Heather Joyce Wolfe

Acknowledgements

"Brevity is the Soul of Wit"... Shakespeare's Hamlet

I have just been reminded of this quotation as I begin to write my "thank yous" and acknowledgements. This part of the book, quite honestly, has been a stumbling block for me. So many people in my heart and mind that I would like to mention who have contributed to this book, to my life and to my wellbeing. Some of you may not even be aware of this. Well, if you have met me, you have had a part – that is how I truly feel, and then you will know who you are, so please acknowledge yourself for whatever part you have played in my life, regardless of how small you may think it is.

However, there are some people I must name, who had an active part in my recovery and in getting this book published – to all of you, more gratitude than I can express.

My 89 years young Mother, Joyce (Wolfe) Ashmore, for her love and support in many different forms – not least of which is her inspiring joie de vivre! She instilled in me love for the Earth and Nature as well as exploration into good health through home grown food.

Other members of my family who have stood by me unceasingly...nurturing, reading, proofing, typing, cajoling, editing, proofing again, persisting, etc. etc. etc... Jess and Noel Walsh, Amber and Poul Walsh Olesen, Heidi Walsh and my Auntie D - Deirdre Wann.

My daughter Anna Krachey; my partner at the time and trailmate, John Ananda; and my friend Susan Kearns, all of whom cared for me with love and commitment after my surgery, beyond the call of duty.

My friend Debra Duxbury, whose persistence in encouraging me to get a biopsy, despite a definitively clear thermography reading, (for which I now know the reason) perhaps saved my life.

My courageous pioneering team of Clairvoyants – firstly my cousin Siobhan Cunningham, whose ability to see inside the body is truly amazing, and who saved me untold anxiety with her accurate perceptions, and to others of similar skill...

Andy and Devita Caponigro, Cheryl Bourget, Margo Mariana, Patricia McCary, Greta Bro, Kedzi Morgan, Angelica Rosemary Adams, Virginia Fidel, Laura Kamm, Susan Pisano, Susan Deren, Flo Aeveia Magdalena, Mary O'Driscoll and Patricia Quinn.

I am very aware of the art that it takes to deliver information in this way, and am extremely appreciative for all of your skill and compassion.

Those people who gave their time to read this book and give me constructive feedback along the way......my nursing friends, Valerie Freeman, Olga Brookes and Ann Pallin, my cousin Dr. Catherine Wann Cullen and also Dr. Martina Glacken Hurley. Invaluable tips from my mother, Joyce Ashmore, and Aunt Deirdre Wann, cousins Jennifer Wann, (for typing too!) Siobhan Cunningham, Mary Dignan and Tina Cunningham, as well as many friends and relatives both in Ireland and the USA – Margaret Larminie, Ella Lowry, Patricia and Michael Quinn, Yvonne Fitzgerald, Barbara Fleming, Claire Fry, Priya, Dorene Palmer, Lainey Ennis, Robin Carroll, Janice Koskey, Elisabeth Bunker, Genevieve Drevet-Miller, Debra Duxbury, Elise DeMichael and Hilary Morgan. Your time, expertise and awareness have made a difference. A special appreciation for Janice, Priya and Hilary for their particular expertise.

Thanks to all those who were on my email list and said prayers, and sang chants – especially Fran and SueRama. So much comfort – thank you. Special thanks to Mirabai Devi for her commitment to my healing, and for her ability to demonstrate the Love of the Divine Mother. To Howard Wills for his Prayers and for abundant kindness, and to Thupten and Chozom Gonpo Hara in India for their unfailing love and prayers, and to Edemir Rossi for his healing hands, words of encouragement and love. For expert teaching, given so humbly, on the healing power of Sanskrit Chant I want to acknowledge Thomas Ashley Farrand.

I want to mention a few people who especially made my life easier along the way.... first in the USA, Thea Fournier for expert nutritional care, Kathy Bucholska for healing hands, Jesse Goldman for impeccable packing, Ruth Bayer for picking up the pieces so well, Donna Caramello for joyful support with my work, Ben Sheppard for webhosting without question, Michael O'Leary for all his kindness, and for his beautiful Irish voice! To Jen and John Newcomer and their children Julia Moon and Benjamin for opening their home (and garage!) so graciously to me during a time of endings and new beginnings.

In Ireland - Marie Conaty, my Irish Anam Chara, in the truest sense of the word, Barbara Fleming, for shelter, wit and awe inspiring kindness. Dorene Palmer, my house mate, for friendship and Divine Food.

Yvonne Fitzgerald, for so much loving support, and Owen Maguire for whizz technological assistance given with great patience and gentleness. Joy Nuzum, for her generous heart and openness to Universal Messages.

Ann McMahon and Bernie Dalton, sisters of mercy and humour at the perfect moment in time! Angels are all of you…..

For abundant love, laughter and harmonious healing in the warm climate of Brazil with John of God ("Miracle Healer") I am so grateful to AnnMaria Dunne, our facilitator, Dave Kenna, Angela Collins and Norah Conway. I want more!

My "oldest" and dearest women friends here in Ireland, Jill Cole, Stephanie Sullivan, Diane Carswell, Barbara Micks, Olga Brookes, Ann Pallin and Valerie Freeman for their constancy, comfort and laughter.

A big thank you to Stevey McGeown, my very dynamic Coach, who moved me out of my "stuckness" to get this book done – time and money so well spent!

I have much appreciation and admiration for the medical staff of Lahey Clinic North in Massachussetts, who showed me genuine caring as well as skill.

Dr. Dermot Rafter and his very efficient office staff have been kind, skilled and wonderful support for me since my return to Ireland. Your openness to my sometimes unorthodox ways, while giving me the conventional care that I required, has been very much appreciated. You made more difference than you may realize.

Last, but not least, to my Book Buddy, my sister Jess Walsh, for her love of flowers and her ability to capture them on camera, as well as her contribution to this book in many different ways. And also to Cari Connors, who as you can see has done such a beautiful job with layout and design.

Heather J

Some notes before reading….

I have taken some liberty with the use of capital letters to emphasise certain words where I thought it was appropriate to bring more attention to that subject. This is the license I gave myself for self publishing!

I realise that I have written this book with the computer in mind, and that not every-one has a computer, or even uses one. I apologise to those people, and suggest that if cancer is a diagnosis, to ask a friend or family member to do the research with them, or for them. This is where a Buddy is invaluable. If you are looking at prevention and exploring this subject and do not know how to use a computer, I would suggest that now is the time to learn. It is a big "learning curve" to begin with, but once that is faced there is a whole new world that opens up in many different ways. I can say this from my own experience. Like anything else that one enjoys, choice and priorities are necessary. Be aware of the effects of spending time in front of the screen and take steps to counteract this. See **Geopathic Stress** and **ELFs**.

With regard to websites, I have mentioned some that have a sales pitch. I don't reap anything from any of these, or sell any products, other than this book and my services. I decided that the information given in the websites that I chose was valuable, and if you buy any products that is your choice. Some of these people will benefit financially, and I am not opposed to that if what they offer is helpful and offered with good intention. I feel the same about the books, CDs and DVDs that I have recommended. Most of them come from my own journey over the years, and some may be older, but the information seems timeless and invaluable. Some of the authors are personal friends and colleagues whom I highly respect, and I wanted to share them with you.

A percentage of the profit from the sale of this book will go towards a fund to help support women diagnosed with breast cancer who want to choose alternative care and do not have the means to do this.

Best wishes on your Journey, wherever it may take you…

HJW

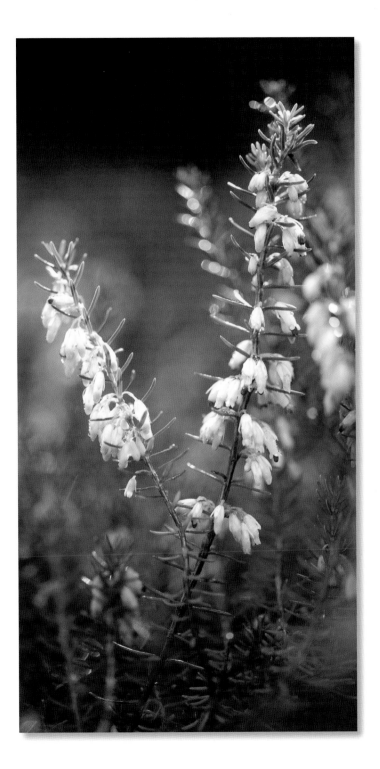

Contents

All disease is an imbalance of the Soul, individually, collectively and globally.

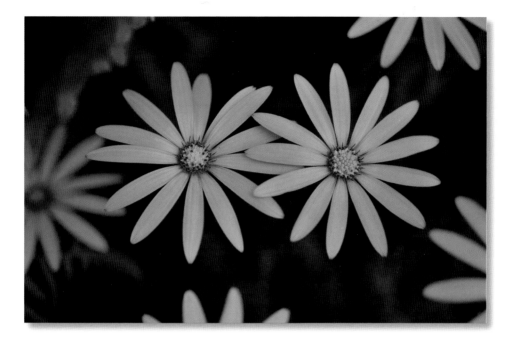

Acceptance, Addiction,
Affirmations, Air, Angels,
Angiogenesis, Apoptosis,
Attention, Attitude

Acceptance

If one can accept, moment by moment, everything that is happening to him or her, life flows and struggle is absent. However, this is a pretty lofty state of Being – one that we are all striving for – living in the present moment. There are many ways to learn acceptance and illness is one way – cancer not being the least of them. If the moment is embraced totally, rather than pushed away, then there is the opportunity for change. Practice makes perfect. Many spiritual paths have guidelines for this practice. This is the core teaching in meditation, which has now been studied and proven to be helpful in many different ways for our health, and even in reversing disease.

Books:
Everything becomes your Teacher -100 Lessons in Mindfulness By Jon Kabat-Zinn
The Power of Now by Eckart Tolle (also audio)

Addiction

Most of us have at least one major addiction. An addiction is a habit or substance that claims our attention outside of ourselves, thus keeping us from knowing our real Self. It can be work, hobby, food, drink, drugs, relationships, TV, movies, video games, exercise or a mental habit that is repeated, to name a few. The definition of an addiction is something that one is powerless to stop, and therefore needs help to change. Some addictions are of course more life threatening than others, but all affect our health negatively in the long run.

Jean Liedloff lived with a tribe in the South American jungle whose society was healthy, with no addictions. She observed that the children were held next to the body of either the mother or father for the early years of their lives, until they had no more need for this. They were also given a lot of freedom and trust of their own knowingness regarding their actions. In other words the Mother Principle was more evident in both sexes than in many other cultures, showing us a healthy role model for balance of the Masculine and Feminine. When human needs are met then the Energy Field of the individual is intact and not lacking. Unresolved trauma and inherited genes play a part in a fragmented Energy Field which gives a feeling of lack.

Where there is a feeling of lack inside this is projected outside in an attempt to fill the gap. This is what we call addiction. Healing occurs when this gap is addressed and filled with this Mother Principle, in whatever form, and by whatever gender has the appropriate way of being to access the gap and the Energy to allow it to fill.

Of course this is not the whole story around addiction. We must take into account our lineage, genes, environment, the company we keep and the addictive nature of that which we ingest, as well as actions stemming from our mental and emotional state. A certain amount of vigilance is necessary to keep aware of how we live our lives. Most of us need help at some time in our lives to correct or avoid addiction.

Books:
The Continuum Concept by Jean Liedloff
Society as an Addict by Ann Wilson Schaef
How to Quit without feeling S++T by Patrick Holford, David Miller PhD
    and Dr. James Braly

Affirmations

An affirmation is a positive statement which helps to change an unhealthy pattern of thinking. Here is one example…

Begin a sentence with the words "I AM" having first thought of a positive intention for yourself. Try the following…

> "I AM CREATING THE PERFECT ENVIRONMENT
> IN MY BODY FOR PERFECT HEALTH NOW!"

Write your chosen affirmation on a card and post it wherever you like, as well as putting it in your handbag, car or workplace. Repeat it as many times as possible during your day. Try 21 days for really good results. Say it out loud sometimes; share it with a friend if you wish. Doing anything for this length of time gives an opportunity to rewire the brain, thus breaking old habits and bringing in the new. Doing this for 40 days is terrific! Both require willingness, commitment and discipline.

Suggestions for affirmations are available at no cost on several websites, if you choose to use a computer.

Combining your affirmations with Emotional Freedom Technique (EFT) will greatly enhance and accelerate the results. Mantra (sounds or phrases) repeated can be used also. Sanskrit from ancient India is known to carry extra power.

Books:
You Can Heal Your Life by Louise Hay
The Secret by Rhonda Byrne
The Power of Intention: Learning to Co-Create your World your Way
 by Wayne Dyer Ph.D.
The Law of Attraction by Esther and Gerry Hicks: The Abraham Material

Cards:
The Present Moment: 365 Daily Affirmation Cards by Louise Hay

CD:
I can do it – How to use Affirmations by Lousie Hay

Websites:
www.emofree.com
www.louisehay.com
www.healingcancernaturally.com
www.vitalaffirmations.com

Air

Oxygen, and the lack of it, is very important in relation to cancer cells. These cells do not live in a well oxygenated body, so make sure that the air you breathe has plenty of it, as free from pollution as possible, as in nature. Remember to open windows whenever possible.

Breathe deeply and consciously several times daily – one minute at a time is better than none, and can work wonders.

If it is possible for you, choose an aerobic exercise at least three times a week, like walking briskly, swimming, biking or dancing. Some yogic breathing will also do the job.

Books:
Kundalini Yoga by Shakta Kaur Khalsa
Energy Exercises by J. Chitty and Mueller

Angels

These days the word Angel seems to be appearing in many different places, though history states that they have always been around. Angels are known to be God's helpers. Apparently at present many are unemployed and would love more opportunities to be of service to humankind. It is said that each of us has a Guardian Angel with us at all times, though most people in this busy world do not listen to the guidance given. However many of us have some experience of what we would call 'Angelic' help at some time in our lives. Apparently Angels do like us to ask for what we want, so why not ask and see what happens? Making note of the results is good affirmation.

Angels are a source of readily available and constant support, whether we believe in them or not.

Book:
Angels in My Hair by Lorna Byrne

Cards:
The Original Angel Cards by Kathy Tyler and Joy Drake
Healing with the Angels (Oracle Cards) by Doreen Virtue, Ph.D.

Angiogenesis

Angiogenesis is the name given to the process whereby a growing network of blood feeds cancer cells or a tumour.

The science of anti-angiogenesis is the attempt to cut off the blood supply that a cancer cell needs for its growth. Diet and/or medications can be very effective.

Books:
Foods to Fight Cancer by Professor Richard Beliveau and Dr. Denis Gingras
How to Prevent and Treat Cancer with Natural Medicine by Drs. Michael Murray, N.D., Tim Birdsall, N.D., Joseph E. Pizzorno N.D., and Paul Reilly N.D.

Apoptosis

Apoptosis is the natural way that our body defends itself against abnormal cell growth, including cancer cells. Various foods, medications and lifestyle can affect this. As we age, apoptosis does slow down leaving us more vulnerable to cancer if we do not pay attention to the things that can keep this process going, such as digestive enzymes, good levels of oxygen, exercise, certain foods, healthy immune system and adequate sleep.

Book:
Foods to Fight Cancer by Professor Richard Beliveau and Dr. Denis Gringras

Attention

Many of us have difficulty paying attention to our own needs, while finding it very natural to give attention to the needs of others. This often leads to resentment as an imbalance in giving and receiving occurs in our energy system. This in turn leads to dis-ease. It serves us well to notice daily how we truly feel and what our needs are - and then to pay attention to meeting them! A 'check-in' with a friend, therapist or coach can often speed up this process and save us much time and trouble.

Exercise - Four Body Coaching
This exercise can be done by yourself or preferably with a friend or Therapist.

Each of our bodies does have needs, and a voice, if we pay attention. This exercise gives us the opportunity to listen to our *physical, emotional, mental* and *spiritual* bodies before they scream at us in one way or another. e.g. dis-ease.

Sit opposite your friend, or sit with yourself.

Close your eyes. Take a few deep breaths and be still. Your friend will ask you to tune into each of your four bodies in turn, beginning with the *physical*. As you hear or sense what each body is saying to you, verbalise this (keeping eyes closed) and your friend will write it down. Repeat this with the other three bodies, ending with the *spiritual*. At the conclusion of the exercise there can be a discussion as to how your needs can be carried out in daily life – the action to be taken – when, where and how. Be sure to write this down.

Make a follow up date to support positive action in carrying out the revelations! One to two weeks is appropriate in most cases. Doing this on an ongoing basis is optimal.

This exercise serves to show us how some parts of our selves are over emphasised and others sadly neglected.

Check this list daily for your own accountability. You may want to rewrite it periodically as changes take place.

If agreed, you can switch roles with your friend and you do the listening and coaching now, or at another time.

Alternatively, find a professional coach or therapist, which may in the long run be the best choice. Most people are very busy these days and can get sidetracked with their own agendas, quite understandably, and follow through can go by the wayside, with disappointment on both sides.

Remember that this exercise can be done quite adequately by yourself – even on a daily basis. Perhaps keep a special journal for doing this. Most people benefit by being accountable to someone else.

Attitude

Our attitude affects our physical and emotional health. It has the ability to empower or disempower us. What we choose to believe affects our ability to overcome illness. It is an acquired skill. Exploring our attitudes and beliefs, and consequent change, can take a lot of courage. It gives us a whole new way to see ourselves and the world. Learning to eliminate a negative attitude and replace it with a positive one can be quite an adventure.

Each thought produces energy, or energy follows thought. If we embrace this idea we would pay great attention to our thoughts. Positive thoughts create positive energy and negative thoughts produce negative energy. It is as simple as that, and yet it can be difficult to change. The subconscious has to be outwitted.

We can choose to create positive vibrations by our words. With practice and repetition we can replace habitual negative thoughts and words with positive ones. A good example is when we are truly thankful for anyone or anything.

Books:

The Secret by Rhonda Byrne
101 Power Thoughts by Louise Hay

Website:

www.gogratitude.com

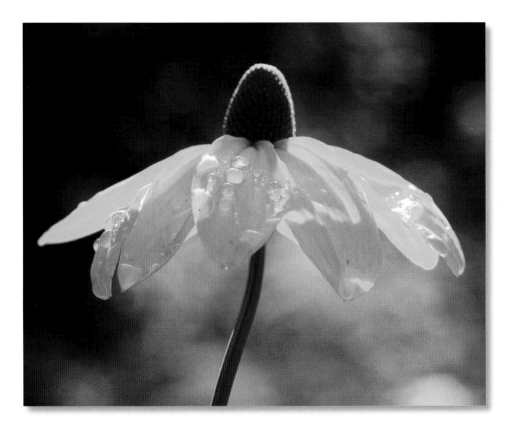

Blessings, Books,
Boundaries, Bras, Breast Care,
Breath, Buddy

Blessings

A blessing is somewhat like giving thanks, and also a prayer, but has a slightly different flavour. Gratitude can be felt at the same time as asking for anything to be blessed. This puts a positive intention around whatever it is – food, a journey, a job interview, the computer, the car, a conversation etc. etc. and gives more opportunity for a positive outcome.

Joey Korn, who uses dowsing as a tool for testing, has created what he calls a Simple Blessing process which is available free to all on his website **www.dowsers.com**

Books

Please ask for the latest edition when buying any of the books below.
Check any book online or on Amazon.co.uk or Amazon.com to find out the content.

Cancer

Cancer Explained by Professor Fred Stephens

The Answer To Cancer Is Never Giving It A Chance to Start by Hari Sharma, M.D. & Rama K. Mishara, G.A.M.S. with James G. Meade, PH.D.

Breast Cancer? Breast Health! The Wise Woman Way by Susun S. Weed

Cancer by Matthias Rath M.D.

An Alternative Medicine Definitive Guide to Cancer by W. John Diamond M.D. and W. Lee Cowden M.D. with Burton Goldberg

How to Prevent and Treat Cancer with Natural Medicine by Dr. Michael Murray, Dr. Tim Birdsall, Dr. Joseph E. Pizzorno, Dr. Paul Reilly

Foods to Fight Cancer by Professor Richard Beliveau and Dr. Denis Gringras

Your Life in your Hands: Understanding, Preventing and Overcoming Breast Cancer by Professor Jane A. Plant Ph.D, C.B.E.

The Key Model: A New Strategy for Cancer Recovery by Dr. Sean Collins, B.A. (Psych) D.C.H. and Rhonda Draper B.A. (Psych) Dip.C.H.

Cancer Recovery Guide by Jonathan Chamberlain

Cancer: Step Outside the Box by Ty M. Bolinger

Cancer-Free:Your Guide to Gentle Non-toxic Healing by Bill Henderson

The Cure for All Cancers by Hulda Clark Ph.D., N.D.

Cancer: Cause and Cure by Percy Weston

Say No to Cancer by Patrick Holford

The Macrobiotic Approach to Cancer by Michio Kushi & Edward Esko

Herbal Medicine, Healing and Cancer by Donald Yance Jr. and Arlene Valentine

Nutrition

Eat to Live – A Phyto Protection Plan for Life by Kenneth Setchell and Sue Radd

The Gerson Therapy: The Amazing Nutritional Program for Cancer and Other Illnesses by Charlotte Gerson and Morton Walker, D.P.M

The pH Miracle by Robert O.Young Ph.D and Shelley Redford Young

Perfect Health: The Complete Mind Body Guide by Deepak Chopra M.D.

Cellular Awakening: How your Body Holds and Creates Light by Barbara Wren

Supplements Exposed: The Truth They Don't Want You To Know About Vitamins, Minerals, and The Effect on Your Health by Brian Clement

Sprouts: The Miracle Food by Steve Meyerowitz

Water: The Ultimate Cure by Steve Meyerowitz

Your Body's Many Cries for Water by Dr. F. Batmanghelidj

The Healing Power of Water by Masaru Emoto

Discover Nutritional Therapy by Patricia Quinn

The Body Ecology Diet by Donna Gates with Linda Schatz

Live Right for your Type by Peter J. D'Adamo N.D. with Catherine Whitney

Foods to Fight Cancer by Prof. Richard Beliveau and Denis Gingras

Food Enzymes - The Missing Link to Radiant Health by Humbart Santillo B.S., M.H.

Prescription for Nutritional Healing by James, F. Balch, M.D. and Phyllis A. Balch, C.N.C.

Dr. Atkins' Vita-Nutrient Solution by Robert C. Atkins, M.D.

Raw Juicing by Norman Walker

Bragg Healthy Lifestyle by Paul C. Bragg N.D. Ph.D and Patricia Bragg N.D. Ph.D.

Prannie Rhatigan's Irish Seaweed Kitchen

The Choice: The Programme by Bernadette Bohan

Wheatgrass – Nature's Finest Medicine by Steve Meyerowitz

Flax Oil as a True Aid against Arthritis, Heart Infarction, Cancer and other Diseases by Joanna Budwig

Fantastic Flax by Siegfried Gursche

The Detox Mono Diet: The Miracle Grape Cure and other Cleansing Diets by Christopher Vasey.

Iodine -Why you need it - Why you can't live without it by David Brownstein, M.D.

The China Study by T. Colin Campbell, Ph.D. and Thomas M. Campbell II

Your Life in your Hands: Understanding, Preventing and Overcoming Breast Cancer by Professor Jane A. Plant Ph.D, C.B.E.

Live Right for Your Type by Dr. Peter D'Adamo

Healing with Whole Foods: Asian Traditions and Modern Nutrition by Paul Pitchford

Eat to Live: A Phytoestrogen Protection Plan for Life by Dr. Kenneth Setchell and Sue Radd

Supplements Exposed: The Truth They Don't Want You To Know About Vitamins, Minerals and Their Effect On Your Health by Brian Clement

Women's Issues and Health

The Wisdom of Menopause by Christiane Northrup, M.D.

The Only Menopause Guide You'll Need by Michelle Moore, M.D.

Sex, Lies and Menopause by T.S. Wiley, with Julie Taguchi, M.D., and Bent Formby, Ph.D.

The Return of Desire by Gina Ogden

Healing Love through the Tao: Cultivating Female Sexuality by Mantak Chia and Maneewan Chia

The Continuum Process by Jean Liedloff

Leaving Abuse Behind by Sarah Daniel

Society as an Addict by Ann Wilson- Schaef

CoDependent No More by Melody Beattie

Co-Dependence: Misunderstood – Mistreated by Ann Wilson-Schaef

The Journey by Brandon Bays

What Your Doctor May Not Tell You About Breast Cancer – How Hormone Balance May Save Your Life by John Lee M.D.

Exercise

Kundalini Yoga by Shakta Kaur Khalsa

Energy Exercises: Easy Exercises for Health and Vitality by John Chitty and Mary Louise Mueller

The Health Benefits of the Rebounder by Albert Carter

Healing Light of The Tao: Foundational Practices to Awaken Chi Energy by Mantak Chia

Wuji Gong by Grand Master Wei Zhong Foo

Da Dao Chan Gong by Grand Master Wei Zhong Foo

Meditation, Mind and Breath

The Miracle of the Breath by Andy Caponigro (CD also)

The Presence Process: A Healing Journey into Present Moment Awareness by Michael Brown

The Miracle of Mindfulness by Thich Nat Hahn (CD also)

Meditation by Sogyal Rinpoche

Letting Everything Become Your Teacher by Jon Kabat-Zinn

The Way of Mastery: Shanti Christo Foundation

The Power of Now by Eckart Tolle

You Can Heal Your Life by Louise Hay

The Law of Attraction by Esther and Gerry Hicks: The Abraham Material

The Secret by Rhonda Byrne

The Power of Intention: Learning to Co-Create your World your Way by Wayne W. Dyer Ph.D.

101 Power thoughts by Louise Hay

Sound Healing

Return to Harmony - Creating harmony and balance through the frequencies of Sound by Nicole Lavoie

The Healing Power of Sound: Recovery from Life-Threatening Illness Using Sound, Voice and Music by Mitchell L. Gaynor, M.D.

Music and Sound in the Healing Arts by John Beaulieu, N.D.

Chakra Mantras by Thomas Ashley-Farrand

Energy and Body Healing

The Power to Heal: A Clear, Concise and Comprehensive Guide to Energy Healing by Robert Pellegrino-Estrich

The Creation of Health: The Emotional, Psychological and Spiritual Responses that Promote Health and Healing by Caroline Myss Ph.D., and C. Norman Shealy M.D., Ph.D.

Wuji Gong by Grand Master Wei Zhong Foo

Da Dao Chan Gong by Grand Master Wei Zhong Foo

Healing Light of The Tao: Foundational Practices to Awaken Chi Energy by Mantak Chia

Quantum Touch by Richard Gordon

The Polarity Experience by Richard Gordon

The Polarity Process by Franklyn Sills

Hands of Light by Barbara Brennan

Tapping your Way to Health by Roger Callahan

Emotional Healing in Minutes by Valerie Lynch

Healing Trauma: Restoring the Wisdom of your Body by Peter A. Levine Ph.D
(also audio)

The Illustrated Encyclopaedia of Alternative Healing Therapies by Jenny Sutcliff

Light - Medicine of the Future by Jacob Liberman, O.D., Ph.D.

Dowsing for Health by Patrick MacManaway

The Pendulum Kit by Sig Lonegren

Dowsing: A Path to Enlightenment by Joey Korn

Medicine Hands by Gale McDonald

Flower Remedies by Edward Bach

Bush Flower Remedies by Ian White

Relationships

Journey of the Heart: The Path of Conscious Love by John Wellwood

Intimate Communion by David Deida

Nonviolent Communication: A Language of Life by Marshall B. Rosenberg, Ph.D.

Men are from Mars and Women are from Venus by John Gray

Miscellaneous

Coaching: The Key to Unlocking your Potential by Carmel Wynne

You Can Heal Your Life by Louise Hay

The Continuum Concept by Jean Liedloff

There is a River: The Story of Edgar Cayce by Thomas Sugrue

Cleaning Yourself To Death: How Safe Is Your Home? by Pat Thomas

*Human Body: An illustrated Guide To Every Part Of The Human Body And
How It Works.* DK (A Dorling Kindersley Book)

Beyond Aspirin – Nature's Answer to Arthritis, Cancer and Alzheimers Disease
by Thomas M. Newmark and Paul Schulick

The Mens Health Book by Dr. Mark Rowe

A Call to Power: The Grandmothers Speak by Sharon McErlane

Your Breasts: What Every Woman needs to Know – NOW! by Brian H. Butler

Faith, Hope and Healing by Bernie Siegel M.D. and Jennifer Sander

Spontaneous Healing by Andrew Weil M.D.

The Tibetan Book of Living and Dying by Sogyal Rinpoche
The Complete Idiot's Guide to the Power of The Enneagram by Herb Pearce
Linda Goodman's *Sun Signs*
Archetypes by Carolyn Myss
How to Quit Without Feeling S++T by Patrick Holford, David Miller Ph.D.
    and Dr. James Braly
Angels in my Hair by Lorna Byrne
Love without Conditions by Paul Ferrini
Silence of the Heart by Paul Ferrini
Anam Cara: Spiritual Wisdom from the Celtic World by John O'Donoghue
The Life You Were Born To Live: A Guide To Your Life Purpose by Dan Millman

Boundaries

Many women have boundary issues. We love to give and often end up giving away too much, creating depletion, resentment and often hopelessness – a good cancer environment. At the same time there is often fear around receiving. The giving can be an addiction to avoid our feelings and keep us stuck. What are we afraid of? This is every woman's quest.

If you have a cancer diagnosis this issue will require much attention during your treatment and healing. This opportunity to expand your awareness is a gift to learn the truth about your needs.

Books:
Co-Dependence: Misunderstood – Mistreated by Ann Wilson-Schaef
CoDependent No More by Melody Beattie
Society as an Addict by Ann Wilson-Schaef

CoDependency Blues **by linde fidorra**
    I've got a special kind of blues
    I live in other people's shoes
    I know exactly how they need to be
    It's called CoDependency.
    I see you have a problem, what's wrong with you
    I bet I can solve it, just give me a clue
    I've read all the books on how to change

I'll help you rearrange.
I just can't bear to see you sad and blue
Let me help, I'll take care of you
No I don't mind, can't you see it's my CoDependency.
Other people have problems while I'm alright
If they listen to me they'd see the Light
I'm in control, I always stand tall
And I don't know myself at all.
I try to fix everybody except myself
My unresolved issues are up on the shelf
I'm starting to wonder who I could be
  without CoDependency.

Bras

The bra that you wear is significant. A bra that is too tight (especially under wired) can constrict the flow of the lymph system in the breast, preventing required nutrients and oxygen to get to the breast tissue, or allowing the release of toxins. This is good ground for breast disease of all types, so pay attention to the comfort or discomfort that your bra provides. There are especially trained assistants in many stores to help you find your perfect bra!

If you have had breast surgery your choice of what is next your skin becomes a priority. There are people and stores knowledgeable in this area. Ask your doctor or nurse. In the end it is you who knows what feels good or not, and you who gets to choose.

Buying a good anatomy and physiology book is helpful, if you don't already have one, to see your entire lymphatic system, and any other part of your body.

Book:
Human Body: An illustrated Guide To Every Part Of The Human Body And How It Works. DK (A Dorling Kindersley Book)

Website:
www.breastcancersupport.org

Breast Care

Any women's clinic or cancer society will be glad to give you a pamphlet on Breast Care Examination.

Ask your doctor, friend, or nurse practitioner for instruction.
Try to do this practice every month, if not every day. The shower is a good venue for this encounter.

Look for changes. If anything worries you please have it checked. This is the key. Watch for change of shape or sensation in breast and nipples, lumps, discharge, skin changes, puckering or dimpling.

A second opinion can be most beneficial.
Pay attention. Share your concerns. Procrastination can be fatal.

Google for instructions:
www.breastselfexam.ca/

Breath

Breath is necessary for life. Most of us need conscious retraining, and release of the muscles that keep our breath shallow.

Exercise, Yoga, Bodywork and Emotional Release Work as well as various methods of Breathwork are some of the ways to accomplish this.

Try **Alternate Nostril Breathing** as follows........this is one variation.

> Sit comfortably with your spine straight.
> You can be on the floor, or in a chair.
> Rest your left hand on your lap with index finger and thumb connected.
> Close the left nostril with the index finger of the right hand.
> Inhale deeply through the right nostril for the count of 8.
> Now close this nostril with your right thumb.
> Exhale through your left nostril to the count of 8, and then inhale again
> through the same nostril again to the count of 8.
> Close this left nostril with your index finger and breathe out through the right,

and breathe in again through the right................

Repeat this pattern for 3 to 5 minutes. You can let go of the counting if that suits you better.

To finish, inhale deeply through both nostrils – hold the breath for a moment or two – then exhale slowly.

Notice how you feel now.

You can also breathe in and out through the left nostril only for a calming effect, (lunar/feminine) or the right nostril only for a more energizing effect (solar/masculine).

This breathing exercise brings in oxygen, balances Blood pH, releases negativity, calms the nervous system and lowers blood pressure. For best results practice this a few times daily, though even once can work miracles! If necessary it can be done in bed, either before rising or before going to sleep.

Books:

The Miracle of the Breath by Andy Caponigro

There is also a CD of the same name to accompany this book.

The Presence Process by Michael Brown

Kundalini Yoga by Shakta Kaur Khalsa

Buddy

If you are diagnosed with breast cancer a Buddy will help you to do the Journey with more ease and less stress.

If you are a woman, a woman Buddy is probably the best choice – regardless of how close you are to a man, and even if he is also your Buddy.

You need a woman buddy, whether for prevention, crisis or healing. Women need women. A helpful hormone is released when women come together, apart from any other reason, and there are many.

We need to receive woman energy back for the woman energy that we give out. Your Buddy will have a total commitment to your wellbeing, without distraction. There are degrees of this, of course, and each contract will be unique. Sometimes this person is a professional, such as a Life Coach, Counsellor, or Nurse Counsellor. Sometimes it can be a good friend or family member with time to devote to you, or both. Expectations need to be considered and discussed here regarding length of time, and how much time etc.

Women and men are different. They think differently, and have different needs, and different ways to share themselves. This is a physiological, psychological and hormonal fact.

You and your Buddy will benefit greatly from writing out a plan and reviewing it weekly. Honest communication is of the utmost importance here.

Your Buddy is the person to whom you are accountable, and not necessarily the person who does everything for you, or your dearly beloved, (if you have one) whose role is nonetheless important in a different way.

Do remember that each person and situation is unique, so the above is merely a guideline to be expanded upon in your own way. If you are following conventional guidelines the medical system can provide much support, both in and out of the hospital. The less travelled alternative route may not have as great a support system in place, and so a Buddy is even more valuable in this situation.

Your Buddy can help you to look at options, as well as help you get organized with your priorities and your daily life, in whatever situation you find yourself.

Try reading, or better still, listening to the audio version of *Men are from Mars and Women are from Venus* by John Gray.

Book:
A Call to Power: The Grandmothers Speak by Sharon McErlane

Notes

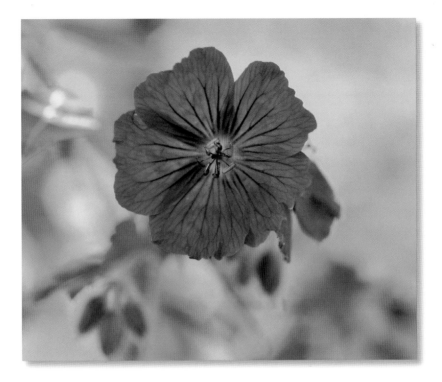

Cards, Causes, Chakras,
Chant, Chemotherapy,
Chewing, Clinics, Clairvoyance,
Coaching, Colour, Commitment,
Communication, Constipation,
Continuity, Counteract

Cards

There are many types of inspirational cards available now in book stores. These can bring you messages of comfort, guidance and strength on a daily basis, as well as feeding your senses with their creative beauty.

Cards:
The Original Angel Cards by Kathy Taylor and Joy Drake
Healing with the Angels Oracle Cards by Doreen Virtue
The Present Moment: 365 Daily Affirmation Cards by Louise Hay
The Irish Fairy Cards by Jaya Moran
The Angel Messenger Cards by Mentor and Merdith Young Sowers
The Healing Cards by Carolyn Myss and Peter Occhiogrosso
The Mother Peace Cards by Karen Vogel and Vicki Noble
The Crystal Ally Cards by Naisha Ahsian
Medicine Cards: The Discovery of Power through the Way of Animals
   by Jamie Sams and David Carsons

Causes

The primary cause of cancer is an imbalance in the cellular chemistry, which has generally been developing over time. Then there is a moment when the cells begin to change and become cancerous. Lack of oxygen, incorrect thinking, feeling, nutrition, compromised immune and hormonal systems, lifestyle and environment, as well as unresolved trauma, can all accelerate these changes. It follows that correction of these can create cell balance, and thus health.

The list below is a general one. When one part is affected the others are consequently also influenced, and so a cycle is begun.

Physical
1. Geopathic Stress
2. Dehydration
3. Lack of nutrients, which can be due to a compromised digestive system, as well as a deficient diet
4. Lack of minerals

5. Acid/Alkaline imbalance
6. Lack of oxygen and toxic Chi
7. Lack of internal and external enzymes
8. Too much food cooked above 43 degrees centigrade (110 F)
9. Lack of essential fatty acids
10. Over-consumption of unnatural fats such as hydrogenated oils, transfatty acids (heated oils) and animal fats
11. Over- consumption of meat, especially red meat
12. Lack of exercise and a sedentary lifestyle
13. Compromised immune system
14. Hormonal imbalance
15. Incomplete absorption of hormones, especially those used in synthetic hormone replacement therapy
16. Lack of phyto-oestrogens
17. Excess mucus forming foods eg., overly-pasteurized homogenized milk and cheese, sugar, refined and processed foods
18. Inflammation
19. Relationship between onset of puberty and menopause
20. Decreased apoptosis
21. Absorption of chemicals and heavy metals through food, air, skin and water eg. aflatoxins, (peanuts) inhaled smoke, radon gas, asbestos, some cosmetics, artificial sweetener, chlorinated and fluoridated water, dioxins from plastic
22. Build up of toxins
23. Lack of regular bowel evacuation
24. Certain parasites and viruses
25. Radiation
26. Wearing restrictive bras
27. Chemicals in antiperspirants
28. Disregard for the rhythm of the body and its needs
29. Over and under exposure to sunlight
30. Free radicals

Mental and Emotional
1. Prolonged stress
2. Unresolved trauma in the brain/cell memory
3. Resistance to personal growth and exploring the subconscious

4. Resentment/anger with oneself or other
5. Conflict/guilt
6. Despair/hopelessness
7. Lack of forgiveness
8. Repeating of old patterns, conscious or unconscious
9. Uncontrolled thoughts
10. Not enough laughter
11. Fear
12. Imbalance in giving and receiving
13. Unwillingness to ask for, or receive, help
14. Inability to receive Love

Spiritual

1. Disconnection from Spirit, the Divine, your True Self/Love causing an imbalance in the Soul
2. Perceived lack of Love – inside and out
3. Lack of true perception and awareness
4. Lack of consistent group spiritual support
5. Disregard for the rhythm of the earth, sun, moon and stars, and the influence exerted by these on each of us

Chakras

This word comes from the Sanskrit word for wheel. It is becoming more widely known that we have seven major wheels (chakras) of energy that act as transformers for the energy between our four bodies - physical, emotional, mental and spiritual. They correspond to our endocrine system and are attached to the spine, both back and front.

During childhood, especially up to the age of seven, these centres are very sensitive and open to suggestion, absorbing the patterns of those around us, as well as forming their own patterns from thoughts and feelings and example. Tears and holes can occur in the chakras along the way from various traumas and life experiences, and if not healed, will cause disease on any level.

N.B. In some systems the breasts correspond to the element of water and free flowing emotional expression, or not, as the case may be.

Books:

The Power to Heal – A Clear, Concise and Comprehensive Guide to Energy Healing by Robert Pellegrino-Estrich

Hands of Light: A Guide to Healing through the Human Energy Field by Barbara Ann Brennan

Chant

Every spiritual path has some kind of chant, which are sounds that are repeatedly said or sung to improve situations, clear the environment and the body, as well as create sacred space.

In this case we are looking at chant as a benefit to our health, and specifically to change the vibration of the body so that it can no longer hold the vibration of cancer. The sounds of the mantras, as they are called, have the power to do this.

Chant has the same kind of guidelines as most medication does. It needs to be done for a certain period of time consistently. Treatment can be effective within two weeks. For more deep rooted problems 40 to 120 days or more, is recommended. There are different types of chant to suit certain ailments, as there are different types of medication. Both can be implemented at the same time.

The optimum number of times to recite any mantra is 108. The significance of this is that the sound of each mantra affects one of the 108 energy points (nadis) connected to the heart. Thus, with this number the heart is charged in a positive manner. There are strings of beads available to help us keep track of the count. They are known as Mala Beads in India.

It is said that mantras work directly upon our karma – those accumulated latencies and tendencies with which we are born. The amount of energy available in our system is increased by these particular sounds. Sound has the potential to either increase or decrease our energy. Many mantras originate in Asia from the Hindu and Tibetan Buddhist Tradition, and could be considered ancient. They are written in Sanskrit, and have stood the test of time.

There are no side effects, except perhaps to purge unwanted energy connected to negative patterns, and to raise our vibration, so that we do not continue in some of our old ways. This is not so bad, if we want to heal! Another side effect could be a feeling of joy, especially if sung in a group.

Search for this in your community. Kundalini Yoga includes chant in its practice. Some music stores carry CDs now, and more are available online.

Book:
Chakra Mantras by Thomas Ashley-Farrand

CDs:
Healing Mantra with Thomas Ashley-Farrand
Health, Healing and Reduction of Karma with Thomas Ashley-Farrand
Prem, or other CD, with Snatam Kaur (Kundalini Yoga)
All is Forgiven by Ashana

Websites:
www.snatamkaur.com
www.ashanamusic.com
www.sanskritmantra.com

Chemotherapy

Chemotherapy side effects can be minimised by good choices. If you do choose to have this treatment it is important to strengthen your immune system and your liver in advance if at all possible. Adding nettles (Tincture or Tea) to your diet is invaluable as they can prevent many common side effects. Dandelion and Milk Thistle are also wonder herbs for cleansing and strengthening the liver. Antioxidants like Selenium, Vitamin C and E encourage the body to secrete more cytokines, natural substances in our bodies which help fight cancer cells (secreted mostly during sleep at night). It has been noted that Folic Acid can help avoid hair loss in some cases.

If you are under conventional medical care please discuss all supplements, herbs and any alternative treatments you may be having with your doctor, to allow for your most comprehensive healing.

A space of three days without supplementation is often advised after your chemotherapy treatment to allow the medication to work fully by itself. Sometimes it is wise to recognize that your Doctor is expert in the field that you are going to him or her for treatment, but may not, as yet, be trained in nutrition or supplementation to avoid side effects. In this case you will have some decisions to make about seeking out someone who may be trained in this area, and sharing this with your doctor.

There is controversy about some supplements, and even foods, counteracting the desired effects of chemotherapy, so knowledge in relation to your treatment regarding this would be advantageous, if you are going this route. There are studies indicating that some nutritional supplementation is better than none, though caution is advised with your choice. Studies are producing new findings on a regular basis.

However, juicing vegetables, especially greens, can be the most beneficial because they are natural foods which are synergistic with your body, and assimilated easily and quickly. Care needs to be taken even with these, and professional advice is suggested, as well as testing the best route for your constitution.

One common side effect of chemotherapy is a suppressed immune system, which counteracts the goal of eliminating cancer cells. While the drug may temporarily eliminate cancer cells, to prevent recurrence an immune enhancing protocol is advisable to help avoid this. Conventional Medicine tends to fall behind Complementary and Alternative in addressing the immune system and nutrition, as prevention is not the focus in most Medical Schools. This is changing in some places, but in the meantime one has to manage one's own care here for optimal results.

Your doctor may be supportive in what you choose, but some may feel safer to stay with what they know. Malpractice is an issue here, as there are rules and regulations within the medical associations. A Naturopathic Physician may be a good adjunct at this time.

The function of the digestive tract is greatly minimized during chemotherapy. This requires attention. Discomfort can be mild with the right support.

Bladder infections are another possibility, and again can be avoided with the correct nutrition, in whatever form you choose.

If antibiotics are necessary, overgrowth of Candida is common and will need some treatment. Probiotics are the number one choice, and can be taken prophylactically, though stronger methods may be required.

Fatigue and "brain fog" are other common side effects which can be minimised by good nutritional support, and ample rest, as well as appropriate exercise.

There are effective alternative medicines to conventional oncology that purport to have less side effects and are less expensive. However these are still powerful "medicines" and require the proper choice and dosage for each situation, as well as supervision and support.

Energy Healing such as Reiki or Acupuncture is often valuable during this time of treatment. Some Chinese herbs are also useful, but must be given by a practitioner experienced in prescribing herbs for your specific chemotherapy drugs.

In addition to all of the above, Emotional Freedom Technique, Affirmations and Spiritual support can speed your recovery greatly.

Books:

An Alternative Definitive Guide to Cancer by W. John Diamond, M.D. and W. Lee
    Cowden M.D. with Burton Goldberg

How to Prevent and Treat Cancer with Natural Medicine by Dr. Michael Murray,
    Dr. Tim Birdsall, Dr. Joseph Pizzorno and Dr. Paul Reilly

Cancer-Free: Your Guide to Gentle Non-Toxic Healing by Bill Henderson

Cancer: Step Outside Outside the Box by Ty Bolinger

The Cancer Recovery Guide: 15 Alternative Therapies by Jonathan Chamberlain

Websites:

www.oncologychannel.com

www.cancerfightingstrategies.com

Chewing

Chewing is extremely important! Watch how you do, or do not, do this. Digestion begins in the mouth with saliva. Indigestion causes toxins which lead to disease.

Make chewing a meditation. See how liquid you can make your food before it goes down to your stomach.

Chewing triggers the rest of the digestive process, as well as relaxing the stomach muscles. It is a gateway to good digestion and assimilation. If you have been a fast eater for a while, changing this pattern takes commitment and perseverance, but is well worth the effort.

You are what you digest, not necessarily what you eat!

Clinics

If you have a cancer diagnosis and want to choose complementary or alternative treatments, or a combination, it is important, and can be life saving, to attend a recommended clinic or hospital, either residentially or as an outpatient. This can be expensive, though some may be covered in part by health insurance, especially those with some orthodox medical supervision. The benefits of doing this is many-fold, including ongoing support and guidelines for treatment with total immersion in making life changes. Below are some suggestions...more will be found in the listed books.

Clinics:
www.pennybrohncancercare.org   (formerly The Bristol Cancer Care Centre)
The Gerson Institute CA. USA **www.gerson.org**
The Simonton Cancer Center CA.USA **www.simontoncenter.com**
An Oasis of Healing, Arizona. USA **www.anoasisofhealing.com**
www.annieappleseedproject.org
Dr. Simoncini, Italy
Mariposas Clinic, Spain

Books:
Cancer Free by Bill Henderson
Cancer: Step Outside the Box by Ty M. Bolinger

Clairvoyance

Clairvoyance means clear sight, and in this case it means the gift of extra sensory perception in the realm of seeing. Different people have the ability to see on different levels. Some can view the organs physically and their state of health or not. Edgar Cayce brought this gift to light in the early 1900s, and is probably the best well known and most documented of all clairvoyants. Dr. Norman Shealy, along with Carolyn Myss, first coined the term "Medical Intuitive" in 1987 as part of their research on intuition and medical application. Often the psychological and energetic pattern is seen along with the physical abnormality, helping the client to understand the cause of a problem, and thus to address it.

Books:
There is a River: The Story of Edgar Cayce by Thomas Sugrue
The Creation of Health: The Emotional, Psychological and Spiritual Responses that Promote Health and Healing by Caroline Myss Ph.D and C. Norman Shealy M.D., Ph.D.

Coaching

A study has been done on Fortune 1000 top executives who invested in coaching for themselves or their company, and it was found that the average return on this investment was 570%. This can also be applied to our personal lives and our health.

Books:
Coaching: The Key to Unlocking your Potential by Carmel Wynne

Colour

Colour Therapy is becoming well known as a healing science, also known as Chromotherapy. Colour is light of different frequencies. Each frequency has a particular resonance that imparts a healing energy. We are surrounded by colour in our environment, and we choose colours of our clothing daily. These all have an effect on us, so if we choose consciously we can bring harmony and healing to ourselves in this very simple and fun way. Our intuition can be a good guide here. Sunshine contains the complete rainbow of colours and as such is a powerful healer, in the correct amount (see *Sunshine*).

It is a well known fact that women generally live longer than men, and also well known that women wear more colour than men, who are often seen in grey, navy, black or brown – the darker colors. Conversely male birds, who often display brilliant colours, live longer than their female companions, who are less colourful. Studies have concluded from this that there is a correlation between the amount of colour that surrounds a body, which can affect health and longevity.

Some cancer clinics are now using Chromotherapy in conjunction with other therapies, with success. Visualisation of a colour going to a specific part of the body, or to the entire energy field, in a meditative state can be a powerful tool for healing.

For example, turquoise is used to stimulate the thymus gland to activate the immune system. A simple light box can be constructed so as to be able to switch panes of coloured glass that shine on the body, or on a specific area.

DVD:
Cancer Conquest by Burton Goldberg

Website:
www.colortherapyhealing.com

Commitment

Commitment to your own healing is an act of Self Love. Most of us, especially when challenged, need someone to be accountable to for optimal success. Intention is the foundation here. Writing what you intend to commit to makes the difference between making it and breaking it. Try it.

Book:
The Power of Commitment by J.W. Von Goethe

> *Until one is commited there is hesitancy, the chance to draw back, always ineffectiveness.*

> *Concerning all acts of initiative (and creation) there is one elementary truth, the ignorance of which kills countless ideas and splendid plans....*

> *that the moment one definitely commits oneself, then Providence moves too. All sorts of things occur to help one that would never otherwise have occurred. A whole stream of events issues from the decision, raising in one's favour all manner of unforeseen incidents and meetings and material assistance, which no man could have dreamed would have come his way.*

> *Whatever you can do, or dream you can, begin it. Boldness has genius, power and magic in it. Begin it now.*

Communication

There are many different ways of communicating. However, as human beings we have been given some extra qualities to bring communication to a high level. We have evolved brains which can send messages to our eyes, ears, vocal cords and muscles to give messages in all sorts of creative ways to our fellow humans, allowing for clear communication and making life more expansive. Most people are not taught good communication, as negative patterns are handed down through our lineage. At this time in history there are opportunities to learn enhanced ways of communicating that can begin at an early age. This is another form of preventive medicine. Holding thoughts and emotions inside produce blocked energy and thus disease.

Book:
Non Violent Communication: A Language of Life by Marshall B. Rosenberg, Ph.D.

Constipation

Constipation is probably the route of all ills. It has many repercussions, resulting from the toxins that ought to leave our bodies through elimination being re-absorbed back into our systems.

Some symptoms of toxicity are allergies, blocked sinuses, skin irritations, haemhorroids, aching joints and a feeling of lethargy and often abdominal discomfort with frequent urination, as the kidneys attempt to remove the toxins.

These are the outward obvious symptoms. Meanwhile there are more effects happening on an inner level that may not be so apparent, such as liver, heart and colon disease, as well as setting the stage for many types of cancer.

One of the major causes of constipation is a magnesium deficiency, due to lack of this mineral in our diet. Magnesium can be found in leafy green vegetables, black beans, pumpkin seeds, nuts, and all whole unprocessed grains – organic if possible. This imbalance of magnesium has occurred first in the soil, due to fertilizers and pesticides used in farming today. Dark chocolate, especially raw, also has an abundance of magnesium. Where these foods are not available green powders can be substituted. The chlorophyll in greens has a molecule which holds the magnesium, making anything green important in this respect.

Magnesium is involved in the synthesis of protein. It reduces histamine levels so is important in the resolution of allergies. It is involved in over 300 functions in our bodies, including hormonal, so a lack of this mineral can be quite serious. It seems that a simple correction in the imbalance of this mineral can make a big impact on a person's health, not the least being the proper elimination of toxins through the digestive system.

Apart from the magnesium dilemma some other causes of constipation can be due to:

A weak adrenal system due to stress overload
An underactive thyroid
Insufficient fibre in the diet, soluble and insoluble
consuming overly acid producing foods
A diet with excessive protein, especially meat
A lack of fluids
Medication
Lack of exercise and poor muscle tone

If constipation has been a problem for you long term. a few simple changes as above may be very helpful, though it can take some time for your body to adjust to your new regime. Detoxification is a side effect and you may feel more comfortable getting some professional supervision with this.

Tips on keeping the lower digestive system moving
1.   Drink several cups of warm water first thing in the morning, followed by a raw apple.
2.   Ensure that your diet includes a sufficient amount of fibre-rich foods, including vegetables and whole grains, if not contraindicated.
3.   Supplement with extra fibre such as oat bran, psyllium husks and/or flax seed, which pull water into the colon, and act as an intestinal "broom".
4.   Avoid dehydration.
5.   A spoon of Aloe Vera juice before each meal works wonders for lubricating the intestines, if not contraindicated.
6.   Some people rely on that first cup of coffee - make sure it's organic, fair trade, fresh and water processed, if decaffeinated.
7.   Try a small glass of prune juice first thing in the morning.
8.   Take probiotics in some form – in capsules if not in fermented foods.
9.   Take some digestive enzymes.
10. Exercise that includes the lower abdomen – massaging the belly in a circular movement from right to left can be very helpful, as well as nurturing.

A note on laxatives

Use sparingly, but these may sometimes be necessary with travel, lack of exercise, faulty diet or digestion, and sluggish liver, not to mention stress. Cascara Sagrada is gentle and less addictive than many other laxatives. Triphalia, an Ayurvedic preparation, is another gentle and effective solution that is less habit forming. Chronic constipation can cause the loss of muscle tone in the bowel and the correct laxative can sometimes help to restore this memory. Colonic irrigation can also help to trigger this mechanism, and is good preventive medicine, as well as very effective detoxification.

One can become dependent on laxatives. This is not necessary.

Check your lifestyle and habits and see your doctor if trouble persists.

Books:
The Body Ecology Diet by Donna Gates and Linda Schatz
Bragg Healthy Life Style by Paul C Bragg, N.D., Ph.D. and Patricia Bragg N.D., Ph.D.

Continuity

This can be difficult, but is so necessary in the healing process, as well as for prevention. Many events can take us off track. Consider finding a Buddy or a Professional Coach and/or a Health Professional to support you in being disciplined and consistent. Our subconscious can be stronger than our conscious mind, so it is useful to be accountable to someone else, and to explore the reasons for our distraction. They may be well buried.

Books:
Coaching: The Key to Unlocking Your Potential by Carmel Wynne
The Key Model: A New Strategy for Cancer Recovery by Dr. Sean Collins,
    B.A.(Psych) D.C.H. and Rhoda Draper, B.A. (Psych) Dip.C.H.

Counteract

If one has a sedentary job to counteract the effects of this lots of exercise is required for balance. Most things in life would benefit from its opposite. Another example would be counteracting electrical stress with time in nature, or balancing intake of acidic foods with alkaline foods. In this way a statement that something is really bad for you can be somewhat negated, rather than a recipe for disaster.

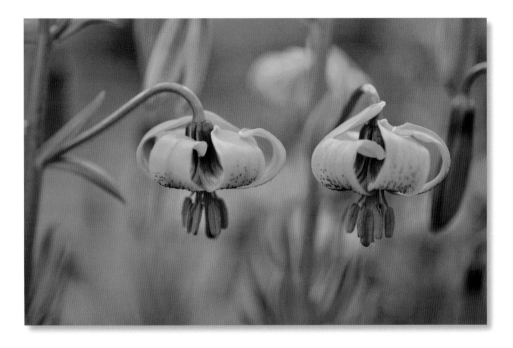

Daily Practice, Dehydration,
Detoxification, Doctor

Daily Practice

Some suggestions might include:

Exercise/Movement/Dance
Conscious breathing
Listening to uplifting music
Meditation and Silence
Sacred Sounds
Singing
Prayer
Angel Cards
Forgiveness
Tapping
Affirmations
Laughter
Journaling
Juicing
Optimal Food Intake
Nutritional Supplementation

Book:

The Key Model: A New Strategy for Cancer Recovery by Dr. Sean Collins, B.A. (Psych.), D.C.H. and Rhoda Draper, B.A. (Psych.), Dip.C.H.

DVDs:

The Choice: Bernadette Bohan
Cancer Conquest: Burton Goldberg
Healing from the Inside Out by Mike Anderson
Cancer Visualisation: Return to Wholeness by Deepak Chopra M.D.

Google:

Breast Cancer DVDs

Dehydration

Our bodies are made up of 70% water, though the brain needs 80%. Dehydration occurs when inadequate water reaches our cells. There are many reasons why we cannot hold enough water to keep our systems healthy. It is easy to presume that because fluid is so readily available that dehydration is unlikely, but the converse is very often true. Not all fluids hydrate our bodies. Alcohol and drinks containing caffeine, (many soft drinks) act as a diuretic and so can cause dehydration. Other reasons are: mental activity, stress, exercise, perspiration, effects of medications, excessive urination and bowel movements.

When we become dehydrated it affects the whole molecular metabolism of the body, possibly causing pain, allergies and asthma, lethargy, headaches, cramps, depression, forgetfulness, high blood pressure, diabetes, dry skin, inflammation, ineffective immune system and destruction of primary amino acids, low oxygen and high acidity. Many of these effects are suitable grounds for cancer.

When we drink enough water it helps maintain the electrical properties of the cells, improves oxygen levels and moistens the lungs, transports nutrients, cushions and lubricates bones and joints, and absorbs shock, regulates temperature, hydrates cells which improves cell communication, removes waste and toxins and empowers the body's healing process. When we become dehydrated the body has a built in protective mechanism where the liver works harder and produces extra cholesterol to protect the dehydrated cells. Conversely hydration creates the correct charge in our system. Essential fatty acids play a major role in helping our bodies hold water, as well as seaweed or a good sea salt with minerals. Potassium and magnesium also play an important part in balancing fluid regulation, found in many foods.

A common suggestion is to drink ½ an ounce of water for every pound of body weight. Other people will say to drink at least 8 glasses daily. Vegetarian diets with lots of vegetables will get more fluid through food than those eating a meat diet.

Books:
Cellular Awakening by Barbara Wren
Your Body's Many Cries for Water by F. Batmanghelidj, MD

Detoxification

Many foods we eat are not digested properly due to a compromised digestive system causing toxic waste products to go back into our system to feed our cells - not optimal for good health. However, if we give time and space to allow these poisons to leave our bodies healing of many diseases can occur, including cancer. Educating oneself about this process makes it easier to understand why we might want to take action.

Chewing our food well and not over eating are good practices to follow to allow for better digestion, and less toxins.

Books:
Cancer: Step Outside the Box by Ty M. Bollinger
An Alternative Medicine Definitive Guide to Cancer by W. John Diamond, M.D. and W. Lee Cowden, M.D. with Burton Goldberg
The Detox Mono Diet: The Miracle Grape Cure and other Cleansing Diets by Christopher Vasey

DVD:
Raw for Life: The Ultimate Experience of the Raw Food Lifestyle

Website:
www.healingcancernaturally.com

Doctor

The Medical Profession has done much research on cancer. The system is set up with a certain structure which can provide support and skilled care for people diagnosed with cancer, as well as those close to them. However this has not been the place to look for prevention, except through various tests such as Mammogram, PET, MRI, Cat Scan, Ultra Sound and more recently the Taylor X trial. These tests do save many lives, if done early enough in someone's cancer process.

Naturopathic Doctors have a more natural approach, but they are less available generally and are often not covered by health insurance.

Some collaboration of treatment could be beneficial to all, as well as more education in medical school on prevention and nutrition.

Books:

Faith, Hope and Healing by Bernie S. Siegel, M.D. and Jennifer Sander

How to Prevent and Treat Cancer with Natural Medicine by Dr. Michael Murray, Dr. Tim Birdsall, Dr. Joseph E. Pizzorno, Dr. Paul Reilly

DVD:

Cancer Visualisation: Return to Wholeness by Deepak Chopra M.D.

Notes

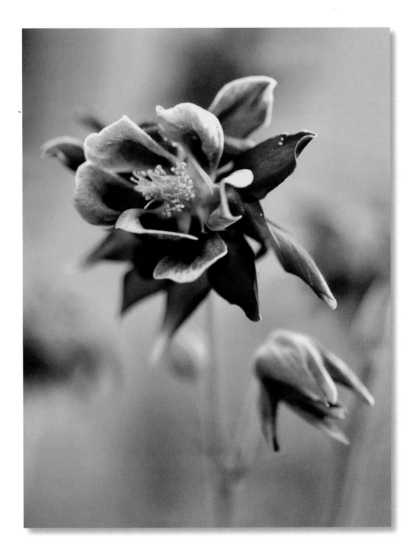

ELFs, Emotions, Environment, Enzymes, Exercise

ELFs

We are surrounded by ELFs - Extremely Low Frequencies - in modern civilization. Everything that plugs in emits a current that is foreign to our own energy system. These fields of extremely low frequency lower our Life Force and can damage our health more than most people realise.

Electric Fields are formed whenever a wire is plugged into an outlet, even when the appliance is not switched on, so it is very important to pull the plug when the appliance is not in use.

There are various products on the market now that can help us counteract the negative effects of ELFs, such as pendants, phone and computer "buttons" and salt lamps to name a few. Going out in nature and breathing pure air deeply are some of the best ways of clearing negative frequencies from our energy fields, as are bathing, showering and swimming.

Placing a cactus and/or a large stick of charcoal near computers, or other technological devices and appliances are two natural forms of reducing harmful rays emitted.

Book:
ELFs by Robert Beckwith

Website:
www.cancerfightingstrategies.com

Google:
ELFs

Emotions

The all important Emotional body ...

In the majority of societies there is repression of the emotional body. Feelings are suppressed, regarded as 'inappropriate' or annoying and time consuming. Those who express their emotion are often regarded as 'rocking the boat', which is not a very comfortable position for either party. However, unexpressed emotion, be it anger, grief, rage, fear or even love, can cause untold harm.

The most common mental/emotional combination in relation to breast cancer is conflict, resentment and hopelessness or despair in some area of life.

For optimal health we all need to communicate our feelings, conscious and unconscious. Seeking professional help is necessary and efficient at certain stages in life.

A cup of tea and a good chat with a friend, or friends, can relieve much distress and tension, and be an adjunct to professional help, though not replace it.

Books:
The Journey by Brandon Bays
The Law of Attraction by Esther and Gerry Hicks
The Presence Process by Michael Brown

Environment

The number one hazard to our health over the past twenty years, in particular the last ten years, is the vibration and content of our environment due to chemical pollution in the air and water, and as a result, in our food.

House cleaning chemicals and synthetic cosmetics are a major cause for concern as we breathe them in and absorb them through our skin on a daily basis. There are now many natural and safe household cleaners and cosmetics available on the market.

Another major source of concern in this regard is the lowering of oxygen in the atmosphere, due in part to industrialisation, car emissions, over-insulated and sealed homes, animal waste gases when over-populated, and the cutting down of the oxygen giving trees in the southern hemisphere.

Time in nature and in water, as well as visualisation and meditation can all help renew and strengthen our life force.

Extremely Low Frequencies are also a major concern. See **ELFS** above.

Book:
Cleaning Ourselves To Death: How Safe Is Your Home? by Pat Thomas

Enzymes

Enzymes are paramount to good health. We have a generous amount of internal enzymes from birth that are like scavengers, helping to digest food as well as toxins and 'rogue cells'. External enzymes also do this, but are only found in food below 120 degrees Fahrenheit. (38-40 degrees Centigrade). If too much cooked food is eaten the internal enzymes get used up, and are often not enough to keep the balance of healthy cells, resulting in disease. We can see from this the importance of including raw food and juices in our diet to eliminate ill health. This also alkalises our blood, which prevents disease inhabiting our bodies.

Fasting on raw food – fruits and vegetables, or their juices, has long been used to cure and prevent illness. Some caution is required with this, and a guide to help you would be advisable, for the first time anyway. The effects of detoxification sometimes need monitoring.

It is also possible, and very often advisable, to take digestive enzymes in capsule form, either before your meal, or sprinkled on your food. There is a formula for ingesting these in a specific time frame that will dissolve the outer protective protein of cancer cells and thus annihilate them. These are known as proeolytic enzymes (see website below).There are also anti-inflammatory benefits to this practice.

Books:
Food Enzymes – The Missing Link to Radiant Health by Humbart Santillo, B.S., M.H.
Bragg Healthy Lifestyle by Paul C. Bragg N.D, Ph.D. and Patricia Bragg N.D., Ph.D.

Websites:
www.hippocratesinst.org
www.cancerx.org

Exercise

This may be the single most important prevention factor for all disease. Be creative.

We have all heard of the many benefits of daily exercise. It reduces heart disease, diabetes and high blood pressure. It controls weight and strengthens bones, muscles and joints. It improves the immune system, while oxygenating the whole body.

Exercise can overcome insomnia, fatigue, loss of muscle tone, poor range of motion, as well as lack of libido.

There has been little talk about the benefits for people with breast cancer until recently. In fact cancer patients were often encouraged to rest and take it easy. Thankfully things have changed over the last few years. Many studies have been done in different countries, and are now showing numerous beneficial effects of exercise for people with cancer.

Regular exercise not only protects against the development of breast cancer, but can speed recovery after any surgery. However the pace and type of exercise is important for each individual. This is where professional help can be necessary.

Many machines are also now available to assist us in strengthening and toning our bodies. Exercise can be done lying down or seated in a chair, if you are unable to do otherwise.

It is good to begin with just a few minutes of exercise daily, if your health is compromised. It is advisable to consult with your health care practitioner, and perhaps get a referral to a Physiotherapist, Personal Trainer or other practitioner in this field if you are recovering from an injury or surgery – and even if you are not!

The psychological benefits of exercise are multitude. It has been shown that it can relieve anxiety and depression. It can even reduce the incidence of secondary cancer, especially breast cancer, as the breasts do not have a large supply of oxygen or nutrients, and need some movement to encourage flow.

A Rebounder is noted as the best exercise devised by man, but great caution should be taken in building up the time you exercise on this.

Please also see **Movement**.

Books:
Kundalini Yoga by Shakta Kaur Khalsa
Energy Exercises by John Chitty and Mary Louise Muller
The Health Benefits of the Rebounder by Albert Carter

Notes

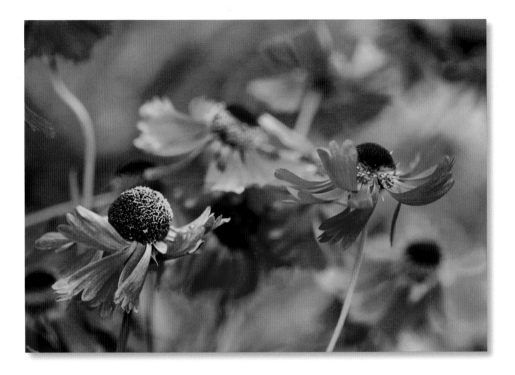

Fats, Fear,
Fibre, Flax, Flowers,
Food Combining,
Forgiveness

Fats

Fat is necessary for our health and survival. However there are good fats and terrible fats. It is imperative to educate yourself about which is which. See **Oils**.

Google: Johanna Budwig for information on her cure for cancer with Flax Oil and Cottage Cheese. She was seven times nominated for her research on Fats/Oils and Health.

Udo Erasmus appears to have the most current knowledge on fats/oils.

Paul Pitchford also has much to share and good guidelines from a mostly Asian perspective.

Books:
Fats that Heal, Fats that Kill by Udo Erasmus, Ph.D.
Foods to Fight Cancer by Prof. Richard Beliveau and Denis Gringras
Flax Oil as a True Aid against Arthritis, Heart Infarction, Cancer and Other Diseases by Dr. Johanna Budwig
Healing with Whole Foods: Asian Traditions and Modern Nutrition by Paul Pitchford

Websites:
www.budwigvideos.com
www.healingcancernaturally.com

Fear

The occurrence of cancer is so prevalent now that almost everyone has been affected by it, and because it is life threatening the word does elicit fear in most people - certainly if it is your own diagnosis, and most likely at times during the challenge of recovery. Dealing with this is a very personal journey. People, in general, are fearful of death, which is the unknown, except perhaps for those who have had near death experiences.

It is important to acknowledge, accept and express fear, if it is there, and then to counteract it in whatever way we choose. This can be a part of ongoing daily (hourly?) practice, and perhaps a large part of the journey of a cancer diagnosis – accepting the moment, whatever it may bring. If we examine fear it is often a projected thought into the future, based on memory of what we have seen or heard in the past. See Attitude.

Emotional Freedom Technique and Thought Field Therapy (Tapping) can be very helpful in reducing fear, and either is quite easy to learn without expense. The only requirements are time and commitment.

Reassurance comes in many forms, not least of which is loving human touch, for which there is no substitute. The presence of another person is very comforting, though time alone to face this fear is part of the growing and healing process, and therefore unique to each person. A Spiritual Counsellor who resonates with your beliefs can help alleviate much anxiety, and bring peace. Verbal expression is imperative for most people, which can include the written word, in person, or via the telephone or computer. Group communication is becoming more prevalent in many forms now. Sometimes the expression of our fears can show us a gift, or a silver lining, and bring some relief.

Books:
When Everything becomes your Teacher by Jon Kabbat Zinn
The Power of Now by Eckart Tolle
Your Healing Hands: The Polarity Experience by Richard Gordon
Emotional Freedom in Minutes by Valerie Lynch

Website:
www.emofree.com

Fibre

A diet rich in fibre can help us avoid many diseases, including cancer. Fibre carries away toxins and cholesterol as well as creating bulk in our intestines, to initiate peristalsis, which consequently moves waste out of our bodies – detoxification in its most natural form. Studies say that fibre contains an anti-cancer property called IP6.

Foods rich in fibre include all legumes, especially green peas, whole grains, fruits and vegetables including their skins, also nuts and seeds, including flax seeds (see Flax). Keep the latter in the fridge or freezer when shelled or ground to avoid rancidity. Eating organically is highly recommended.

We need soluble and insoluble fibre. Many products are available in pharmacies and health food stores. Choose carefully.

Flax

Flax Seed (also known as linseed) as a food has many excellent properties and is easily obtained as either golden or dark brown seeds. Organic is best of course to avoid any chemicals that your body will have to process.

Flax contains lignans which have potent anti-cancer effects both for prevention and treatment of breast cancer.

Flax contains phytoestrogens which will take up the space in the body which more harmful unnatural oestrogens (xenoestrogens) may fill, now known to cause breast cancer in particular.

Omega 3 oils are abundant in flax, important for many areas of our health.

The amount of flax seed or oil to take is an individual decision, especially if cancer is a diagnosis, and opinions differ. Seek professional advice if this makes you feel more comfortable. Two to four tablespoons of flax oil or meal daily, or alternate days, is the amount often recommended. Beginning moderately and increasing the amount slowly can be a good idea. There are some contraindications to taking large amounts of flax, and some people say that taking it for six weeks with a six week break is the best way to deal with this. Finding a method of testing for your own particular dose is probably the most advisable.

Flax seeds can be ground and put on cereal or other food, including soups, as well as baked goods. A coffee grinder works well. It can be taken first thing in the morning on an empty stomach after steeping for fifteen minutes in hot water. This is a chewable drink! It will be mucilageanous and coat the intestines with this healing substance.

Flax is rich in fibre and provides bulk for the intestines, though plenty of water needs to be consumed as flax absorbs a lot of fluid to make this bulk.

This is a good food to research for yourself and then make your own decision about it, with help if necessary.

It is important not to use so much flax that one becomes deficient in other oils that are also necessary for optimum health. Many seeds and nuts contain valuable nutrients that will help prevent disease.

Books:
Fantastic Flax by Siegfried Gursche

Flax Oil as a True Aid against Arthritis, Heart Infarction, Cancer and Other
    Diseases by Joanna Budwig
Fats That Heal and Fats That Kill by Udo Erasmus
Healing With Whole Foods: Asian Traditions and Modern Nutrition
    by Paul Pitchford
The Wisdom of Menopause by Christiane Northrup M.D.
The Body Ecology Diet by Donna Gates and Linda Schatz

Website:
www.bodyecologydiet.com

Flowers

Flowers are God's way of smiling at us.

Their essence can be distilled and given as medicine for the body, mind and spirit. You can learn about this yourself, or seek the help of a trained Flower Essence Practitioner.

Dr. Edward Bach was the modern originator with Bach Flower Remedies. There are now other varieties from many parts of the world.

Flowers bring such beauty into our lives. Their colour is also a major healing factor. Take advantage of the abundance of this gift from Mother Earth.

Books:
Flower Remedies by Edward Bach
Bush Flower Remedies by Ian White N.D.
The Flower Messenger Cards by Meredith Young Sowers

Food Combining

Proteins, Carbohydrates and Fats all require different mediums and digestive juices for optimal absorption. Our modern western diet mixes large quantities of protein and carbohydrates together. The stomach naturally gravitates to producing an excess of acid in this circumstance, to digest the protein. However, carbohydrates require an alkaline medium, so there is somewhat of a struggle for the best digestion.

Over the years this internal confusion takes its toll, resulting in ill health from undigested and putrefied molecules, which produce potent poisons in our system. A larger amount of our internal digestive enzymes are required for the extra digestion that constant improper food combinations elicit. This produces more work for our liver and lymph system to cleanse the toxins produced by incomplete digestion, as well as decreasing our ability for scavenging abnormal cells.

Consequently it makes sense if we are ill, and have a compromised digestive system, that separating our food categories will give us optimum absorption, and thus the chance for better health. Taking digestive enzymes in supplement form is sometimes a good addition, especially in the case of a cancer diagnosis. Guidance from someone with knowledge of this subject is optimal here.

Some rules you may want to pay attention to are as follows:

Eat fruits separately or before meals, because they digest very quickly, and can cause putrefaction if held up by other foods.

Melons ought to be eaten alone, and preferably in the morning.

Eat a small salad before your meal.

Eat one protein at a time, and combine with non-starchy vegetables.

Eat grains and starchy vegetables with low starch or sea vegetables.

Make dessert (natural sugars) a separate meal.

Be conscious of when you are feeling that you have had enough food, (before that full feeling) and stop there. Leaving space for digestion, and some fluid, is important.

In other words, simplify your diet.

Book:
The Body Ecology Diet by Donna Gates and Linda Schatz

Website:
www.bodyecology.com
www.cancerx.org
www.hippocratesinst.org

Forgiveness

All there is is letting go - forgive, forgive, forgive…not to do so hurts us mostly. Holding grudges creates disharmony, resentment and disease. Most of us need help with this one.

Ultimately we will find that it is ourselves who need to change. Much time is wasted in blaming others, and thus being in a victim mode. However it is difficult to rise above this, and so professional help is a good idea. Keeping a journal is an excellent way of becoming more aware of ourselves and our thoughts, so that we can have more choice in our future thinking, and thus feeling.

Books:
Unconditional Love by Paul Ferrini
The Way of Mastery Shanti Christo Foundation
The Journey by Brandon Bays

Websites:
www.radicalforgiveness.org
www.howardwills.org

Notes

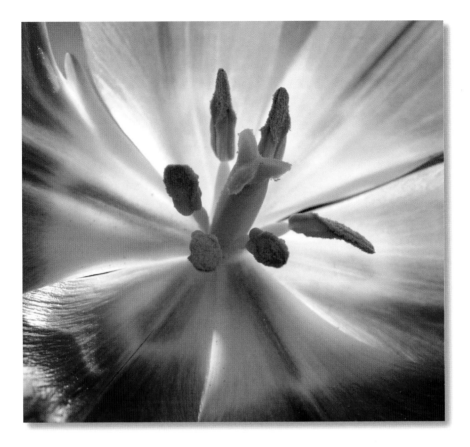

Geopathic Stress,
Grace, Gratitude,
Greed, Groups

Geopathic Stress

Geopathic stress occurs when the natural vibration that comes up from the Earth is distorted by weak electromagnetic fields. It can be caused by fault lines, underground cavities and from certain streams of water, as well as from the effects of our modern lifestyles with its use of electricity and technology, including cell phone masts and microwaves. Radon gas is also a culprit.

As it is unlikely that we will give up much of this lifestyle, or move house, it is advisable to check our homes for the amount of geopathic stress that is in our environment, and counteract it as best we can. There are people who are expert in this field. The position and location of our bed can affect our health greatly.

A study of 175 families of Gypsies, or Travelling People, showed a very low incidence of cancer. They are never in one place long enough (approx. 3 weeks) to absorb the harmful effects of geopathic stress, if it is there. This suggests that cancer is related to location, or from a broader perspective, to the effects of Energy on the human system. Other factors with this group of people may be their thought processes and the level of support within their community life, as well as their organic connection with animals and the natural world.

There are products available to counteract this geopathic stress, should it be a problem for you. Most people these days will find that it will be beneficial to use some kind of protection. Exercise can counteract a substantial amount of stress of any kind, including geopathic. See Environment.

Joey Korn, an American Dowser, states that he loves ELFs, and suggests switching any negative effects from them with a Blessing, as follows:

"If it be Thy Will, may the Powers of Nature converge to increase and enhance the beneficial energies and balance any detrimental energies radiating from this computer, (or other device) for our family, our friends, our pets and for all of benevolent life, for now and into the future, for as long as is appropriate, in deep gratitude. Amen."

This Blessing suggests an invocation to a Higher Consciousness, so if this resonates with you, you may want to insert a Name.

Joey tests the effect of words by dowsing. You could create your own blessing, and check it, or have it checked also.

Books:
Dowsing for Health by Patrick MacManaway
Dowsing: A Path to Enlightenment by Joey Korn

Websites:
www.transformation.net/coils/gypsy.html
www.earthtransitions.com/Earth-Healing/Geopathic-Stress-Q-A.html
www.alternative-doctor.com/geopathicstress
www.britishdowsers.org
www.AmericanSocietyofDowsers.com
www.dowsers.com

Grace

Regardless of who you are, what you have done, or what your diagnosis or prognosis is, there is always Grace. This is similar to Mercy, and does not have to be earned. It is a gift, and goes beyond time and the rational mind. It is yours for the asking – do remember to ask for it. Ask God, Your Higher Self, Divine Mother, Holy Spirit, the Angels or whomever or whatever you might find helpful.

Each situation for each individual is unique.

Please check with yourself if you get what you need and want, such as complete healing, that you are willing to take responsibility for the change in your life? This could be a new level of work or service and more connection with your Soul to speak your Truth.

Take time to listen to the answers when you ask - perhaps write them down.

Gratitude

The practice of being grateful, or giving thanks, is invaluable, beginning first thing in the morning, and throughout the day whenever you choose. This puts your energy system in a "positive spin", the way to healthy cells.

Giving thanks last thing at night promotes restful sleep. Writing a list can give extra benefit.

Remember there is a silver lining to everything - look for it.

Website:
www.gogratitude.com

Greed

Every section of society appears to have the element of greed, however hidden. Be aware. Question motives.

Books:
Society as an Addict by Anne Wilson Schaeff
Sex, Lies and Menopause by T.S. Wiley, with Julie Taguchi, M.D.,
    and Bent Formby, Ph.D.

Groups

Group support seems to be a human need, which is not to say that we do not require alone time. Our gut and heart will tell us which we need and when, if we listen. The Energy of the group seems to dissipate after seven days, so something weekly is optimal in normal circumstances, and perhaps more often if in a crisis situation. The infrastructure of the hospital can be seen and felt as a group, as the team approach is offered with most illnesses. However the physical is paramount here, and the mental, emotional and spiritual dimensions are of equal importance and need attention at all times for balance and healing – most particularly if disease has surfaced (see **Four Body Exercise** under **Attention**).

Churches through the ages have provided much support, solace and structure for many, and still do. Families and societies can do this also, or any group of friends. At this time in history the internet provides support with a few clicks for just about anything! Use discernment with your choices, and protect yourself from computer waves (See **Environment**).

We are in an age where the shadow side of each of us, our families, and all organisations are being brought to light for healing, and as this happens, there is fear, hurt, blame, judgement, grief and loss for many. Look for that silver lining and take the opportunity to move from victim to spiritual warrior. Discover your own truth with gentleness and compassion.

It is important to feel supported in whichever group you find yourself, whether it be an art class, a movement class, a church or a therapy group. There are other choices if not. You will have different needs if you have a cancer diagnosis, and even these will change at each stage of your journey. There are places to meet your special needs at any time. Trust that they will find you.

Ask to see the Social Worker, and check your local community notice boards, for example, grocery stores, doctor surgeries, health centres, health food stores, churches and colleges – and of course Google!

Websites:
www.irishcancersociety.ie
www.actionbreastcancer.ie
www.mariekeatingfoundation.com
www.ark.ie
www.AmericanSocietyofDowsers.com
www.dowsers.com

Notes

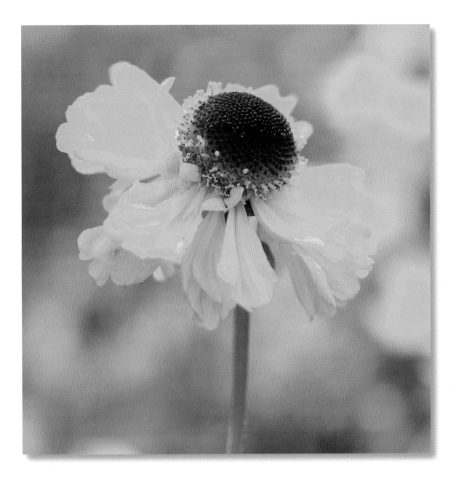

Healing Therapies,
Hormones

Healing Therapies

Our Essence is Love, Light and Sound which come from our Source/Creator/Sun. We need to absorb Light to be healthy. A lack of it creates an imbalance. We can give it out and receive it as transmitters of electricity. If the wiring is faulty due to imbalance or overload, corrections need to take place, often in the form of grounding. One person can help another come into balance by transmitting their Light through their hands or energy field. It is a form of healthy radiation. Perhaps this will become more a part of the medicine of the future?

Therapies such as the following are often helpful:

Reiki, Polarity Therapy, CranioSacral Therapy, Acupuncture, Chakra and Aura Balancing, Crystals, Quantum Touch, Therapeutic Touch, QiGong Healing, Bio Energy Healing, Massage, Shiatsu, Rolfing, Reflexology, Osteopathy, Chiropractic, Jin Shin Jytsu, Jin Shin Do, Unlimited Bodywork,

Sound Therapy, Psychotherapy, BioDynamic Psychotherapy, Hypnotherapy, Colour Therapy, Emotional Freedom Technique (EFT), Thought Field Therapy, (TFT) Kinesiology, Dowsing, NLP and Hypnotherapy.

Google for any of these in your area, or ask at your nearest health food store for local practitioners.

Books:
Quantum Touch by Richard Gordon
The Illustrated Encyclopaedia of Alternative Healing Therapies by Jenny Sutcliff
Medicine Hands by Gale McDonald (Massage for Cancer)

Hormones

Hormones regulate much of our body. However, they in turn are regulated by our thoughts, gender, lifestyle, food and environment.

Oestrogen is a subject of much research and controversy regarding breast cancer. How it is absorbed and broken down in the body is possibly more important than what we actually take into our bodies. Cruciferous vegetables, such as broccoli, cabbage, brussel sprouts and kale are very important in this process of proper absorption, as well as in anti-cancer activity. Fresh is vastly superior to frozen because of the heat needed to blanch the frozen vegetables. Lightly cooked and thoroughly chewed fresh produce is optimal. These foods help to cleanse the liver also, which is where oestrogens are processed in the body.

Supplements with isolated and concentrated phytochemicals are now sold for the purpose of anti-cancer properties, as well as correcting oestrogen absorption. A supplement called Calcium D-Glucarate is a known detoxifier for the body, and in particular for oestrogens. This subject continues to be on the table for examination.

Phytoestrogens found in plant substances such as soy and flax act differently and more naturally in the body than synthetic oestrogens, and can counteract the formation of cancer cells. Soy products have been toted as a health food, but research has shown that this is not always the case, so caution needs to be taken when adding them to your diet. Google dr.mercola soy. Fermented soy foods such as miso, tempeh and natto are the whole form of this bean, and so are superior. As always, knowing the source is a good idea.

The root of the Maca plant from Peru is a staple in South America to regulate hormone balance. This apparently converts to Progesterone in our bodies, which in turn triggers our healthy oestrogen production.

Educating yourself, and finding an informed practitioner before taking any substance which is a known hormone regulator or producer pays dividends.

Women will often opt for this route to alleviate the discomfort of menopausal symptoms, such as hot flushes. In fact hot flushes are one avenue of apoptosis to kill potential cancer cells at this vulnerable time in a woman's life.

If hormonal supplementation is your decision it is a good plan to find a doctor who specializes in bio-identical HRT (hormone replacement therapy) and will test your blood for your specific dosage on a regular basis. This testing can be augmented by other types of testing such as kinesiology, dowsing and/or clairvoyance, depending on your preference, health insurance and your budget.

In preventing Breast Cancer it is important to realize that we are surrounded by unhealthy petro-chemical based xeno-oestrogens. These are in car emissions, (air) cosmetics, (parabens, butyl, ethyl, mineral oils) plastics (especially cling film/ saranwrap) and pesticides. Ingesting sufficient phyto-oestrogens, approximately 15,000 mg daily, is advisable. Fermented soy products, flax meal or oil are the top foods in this category. These compete for the same oestrogen receptor sites in the body, and if there are enough of them they will fill these spaces, rather than the unhealthy oestrogens.

If a diagnosis of oestrogen-receptive breast cancer is found, orthodox medicine will often wish to prescribe medication such as Tamoxifen or Arimadex and other newer drugs to stop the production of oestrogen in the body altogether. Some side effects are a concern. Some studies show that soy and/or flax can supplement the effectiveness of the above drugs, and perhaps prevent some of the side effects.

Doctors and patients are often innocent victims of misinformation. More research here could improve women's health greatly, and save lives.

Books:

Breast Cancer? Breast Health! The Wise Woman Way by Susun S. Weed
The Wisdom of Menopause by Christiane Northrup, M.D.
What Your Doctor May Not Tell You About Breast Cancer – How Hormone Balance May Save Your Life by John Lee M.D.
Sex, Lies And Menopause: The Shocking Truth About Synthetic Hormones And The Benefits Of Natural Alternatives by T.S. Wiley, with Julie Taguchi and Bent Formby, Ph.D.

Websites:

www.breastcancer.org
www.susankomen.com

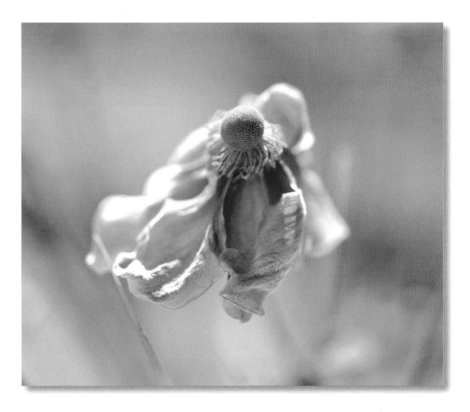

Immune System, Inflammation, Insurance, Intention, Iodine

Immune System

Cancer cells would have a more difficult time developing if the immune system were in top working order. Apoptosis (see **A**) is part of this system, as is our lifestyle and thinking. Unfortunately, there are many things working against it, even in utero through mother's breath, blood and lymph. It is said that over two hundred chemicals have been found in placentas at birth.

See **Treasures**.

The good news is that there are products to remove these safely and quickly, though generally not known in orthodox medicine.

Livers of people young and old need energy for things other than detoxifying chemical pollution! Otherwise chronic fatigue syndrome, environmental illness, fibromyalgia, cancer and a host of other illnesses will present themselves.

One of the best immune defenses is given to us from our Mother through the process of breast feeding, though many people have excellent health without this as there are always many other factors involved.

Medicine in different parts of the world, including Ireland, is exploring how the immune system can be coerced into eradicating breast cancer cells. The cost so far is prohibitive.

Immune System Boosters
> Sunshine
> Happiness
> Laughter
> Affirmations
> Whole Foods
> Raw Vegetable Juices
> Echinacea
> Anti Oxidants
> Mushrooms
> Astragalus
> Aloe Vera
> Selenium
> Phytochemicals
> Seaweeds/Minerals
> Probiotics
> Rebounding

Check out your health food store – different products support different parts of the immune system, and there are combinations. Keep as near to nature as possible. Seek the advice of a health practitioner knowledgeable in herbal medicine before ingesting.

Books:
Breast Cancer? Breast Health! The Wise Woman Way by Susun Weed
The Wisdom of Menopause by Christianne Northrup M.D.
An Alternative Medicine Definitive Guide to Cancer by W. John Diamond, M.D.
    and W. Lee Cowden, M.D. with Burton Goldberg
Spontaneous Healing by Andrew Weil M.D.
An Alternative Medicine Definitive Guide to Cancer by Burton Goldberg

DVD:
Cancer Conquest by Burton Goldberg

Google:
Mantak Chia: YouTube

Inflammation

It is commonly known now that inflammation is a precursor to some cancers, especially long term. Some of the causes include allergy and food sensitivity, fungus, bacteria, viruses and parasites, as well as injury, lifestyle and diet, so it is advisable to pay attention to these and do what is necessary to improve what you can as soon as possible, though this can be a fairly long term process. We must not forget the emotional and mental issues which may be causing the inflammation. Various tests are helpful, and will be different in Conventional and Complementary Medicine. One can affirm the other, or in some instances one will show what the other will not. Finding a practitioner trained in both fields is optimal.

Studies have shown that taking an aspirin a day reduces the incidence of cancer by 45%. However there is the risk of bleeding with this method. Green Tea also contains salicylic acid in its natural form. Herbs containing curcumin, such as tumeric and ginger have also been noted as anti-inflammatory. Some essential oils can also be very effective, such as thyme and rose.

Most anti-inflammatory substances, whether natural or synthetic, are known as

COX-2 inhibitors. COX-2 is largely the culprit in the inflammatory process.

Book:

Beyond Aspirin – Nature's Answer to Arthritis, Cancer and Alzheimers Disease
by Thomas M. Newmark and Paul Schulick

Insurance

Sometimes it may seem that a big chunk of our income goes out on insurance of one kind or another - car, house, health and life insurance, with nothing coming back. However, the nature of insurance is such that if one needs it there it is, and if you don't, someone else is benefiting from your input. Give thanks either way.

Health insurance has many benefits, often covering physiotherapy, counselling, chiropractic care, acupuncture, massage, nutritional counselling as well as other medical services. It may benefit you to find out your full coverage. Call the number on your card or insurance letter, or ask someone else to do it for you - or go online. Look out for free or voluntary services too.

If your income is low, or you are over a certain age, or suffering from certain illnesses or a disability, you may qualify for some kind of health insurance, or assistance, depending on your location.

Part of our insurance is educating our selves in the best ways to avoid illness and have optimal health.

Intention

Energy follows thought – please refer to **Attitude** under **A**.

Each day what is in our mind shows itself, whether at that time or later, as our thoughts create our reality. Taking time to get clear about our intention for anything helps to keep us aligned with our goals and moving forward positively in our lives on all levels. The fuzzy places in our thought processes are often cause for seeking help from a friend, psychotherapist, coach or other practitioner. This decision can make the difference between health and illness and even life and death. The subconscious, as well as the conscious, must be brought into the conversation ultimately.

Book:
The Power of Intention: Learning to Co-Create Your World Your Way
by Wayne Dyer

Book and Audio:
The Law of Attraction by Esther and Gerry Hicks – The Teachings of Abraham.

Book and DVD:
The Secret by Rhonda Byrne

Iodine

Iodine has been found to be lacking in a large percentage of breast cancer cases. Dr. David Browenstein in his book "**Iodine – Why You Need It, Why You Can't Live Without It**" says breast cancer is not caused by a deficiency of chemotherapy, radiation and surgery. "I have no doubt that iodine deficiency, coupled with the increased toxic load of our environment, is a major part of the reason why we have an epidemic of breast cancer." This statement may have a large amount of truth.

Iodine is needed by different parts of the body, primarily the thyroid gland, with the breasts, brain and eyes coming up behind this. If there is only enough for the thyroid then the others do not have their needs met.

The RDA for iodine is 150ug, but many cultures ingest much more than this with beneficial effects.

Each person has unique requirements.

BROAD TEST FOR IODINE DEFICIENCY
Dip cotton ball into tincture of iodine (available at the pharmacy or online).
Paint a one inch circle on soft skin (inner thigh).
If the stain disappears in less than an hour you are deficient.
If the stain remains for more than four hours you have sufficient iodine.

Discuss this with your doctor or other health care practitioner, especially if taking other medications. You may want to share Dr. Brownstein's book with him or her.

Women in Japan who eat lots of seaweed and fish have a very low rate of breast cancer. Men also have a lower rate of prostate cancer, the breast and prostate having the same type of tissue. You can get your required intake of iodine for your thyroid gland by including seaweed in your diet daily. Seaweed also has a substantial amount of calcium in absorbable form, and in fact contains ten to twenty times the amount of minerals that are in land vegetables.

Kelp, wakame, nori (sushi), arame, dulse and carrageen moss are some of the available types of seaweed. It is now known that wakame is particularly beneficial for preventing breast cancer. Natural sea salt from a good source will add a small amount too. Both are available from health food stores and speciality Asian stores.

Some seaweed in the pot while cooking beans in any form removes gas producing effects, and makes the nutrients more available.

Too much or too little iodine can have quite a dramatic effect on your body, as can having enough. Testing for the correct amount is advisable whether through orthodox means, dowsing, kinesiology, or all three.

Too many raw cruciferous vegetables can suppress the thyroid, so this must be a consideration if one is opting for a completely raw diet. Soy isaflavones (genistein) can also have this effect, so moderation is key, as well as considering your own unique needs. As soy is becoming more popular as an antidote to breast cancer with many women, this is worth noting. What is actually being suppressed is the enzyme thyroid peroxidase which is responsible for adding iodine onto the thyroid hormone. Cooking reduces this action, so a balance is important for each individual in relation to the thyroid. Soy milk and tofu are both raw products. If there is the problem of hyperthyroidism these foods can help to naturally decrease the amount of hormones being produced by the body. If medication is being taken it would be important to look at your food intake – food is medicine too.

Speak to your health practitioner about this if you are in doubt, and perhaps keep up with the current research yourself.

Books:
Iodine – Why You Need It And Why You Can't Live Without It
    by Dr. David Browenstein
The Macrobiotic Approach to Cancer by Michio Kushi
Prannie Rhatigan's *Irish Seaweed Kitchen*

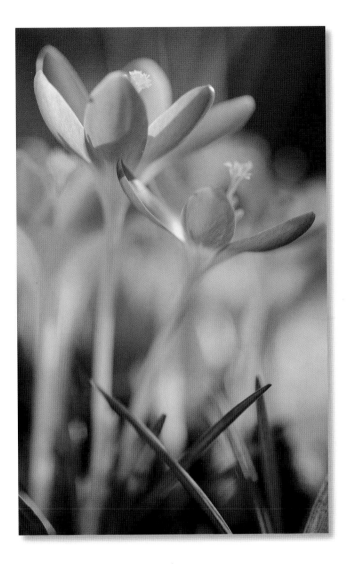

Journal, Joy, Juices

Journal

This is an excellent way to be your own therapist with time the only cost. Write letters to important people in your life to clear any issues which may be weighing you down. To mail or not to mail is your choice. Ask yourself the purpose of mailing. Keep the focus on your own healing.

Very often the act of venting your feelings in this way is absolutely all that is necessary to allow you to move on. The first draught is often better saved a while and rewritten! Each day may bring new insights.

Letters to your self are wonderful too. You can be creative and one part of you can write to another – e.g. the healthy part might have a conversation with the unhealthy part, as in the immune system speaks to the cancer cells?

Just try it and see what transpires.

Joy

Whatever state of health, time of year or life, it is beneficial to everyone to be in a state of joy as much as possible. This radiates from one to another, and around the world, as a positive vibration. What brings joy to one person may be different for another, so spend some time exploring what brings you joy and learn to cultivate it. Ultimately it comes from inside, but it can be stimulated by anything outside, every single moment – difficult in times of challenge.

It is possible for one part of you to feel joy, while another simultaneously feels sadness. The trick is not to obliterate the good feelings with the less positive ones for too much of the time. Taking time for laughter, however fake, will have a healing effect on all of your cells.

Cancer can manifest when the expression of our joy is suppressed.

Book:
The Law of Attraction by Esther and Gerry Hicks – The Teachings of Abraham.

Website:
www.yogalaughter.com

Juices

Juice of fruits and vegetables enters the system very early in the digestive tract, because they have no fibre to be digested to slow down the process. The cells are fed optimal nutrition very quickly and the enzymes in the juices digest abnormal cells and other unwanted materials in the body. Perhaps one of the greatest benefits is the alkalinity that raw vegetable and many fruit juices produce. Some caution is needed with the amount of carrot juice taken due to its high Vitamin A and sugar content. Actually more Beta Carotene is absorbed by the body from cooked carrots than raw, but there are different benefits from the raw form. Both have good properties. Despite the fact that juice is liquid, it is advisable to "chew" it, to allow saliva to mix with it, and also to allow some absorption through the mucous membranes of the mouth. A variety of vegetables and fruits is advisable, though the majority should be vegetables. Do not mix fruits and vegetables, though apple is compatible with most vegetables. Ginger and garlic are very good additions to any vegetable juice. If you have a diagnosis of cancer the level of sugar you ingest, even in juices, needs monitoring, as cancer feeds on sugar.

Remember that orange juice is acid forming and lemon is alkaline forming. Mixing some lemon with the orange can lessen the acidifying effect, unless you want to be more acid, and sometimes that balance is needed. If we listen to our bodies we will know what we need and when. This takes some practice.

Some juicers are more efficient than others, extracting more nutrition e.g. a Titrator or Masticator is more efficient (and more expensive) than a centrifugal juicer. The optimal way of obtaining your daily juice is to do it at home using organic fruits and vegetables. Juicing with any machine is better than nothing at all. Individual needs vary. Hand operated juicers are also available, at least for wheatgrass.

Owning a juicer does not make juice!

If you "haven't time" to juice I highly recommend taking a supplement daily that has at least 13 fruits and vegetables. Much research has been done on this. Plants contain the energy of the sun as well as enzymes and phytochemicals, all of which we need.

However you do it, juices (phytochemicals and antioxidants) are a great insurance against cancer (and it's re-occurrence), heart disease, diabetes and almost every other disease.

Please be aware that too much raw cruciferous vegetables (the cabbage family) do affect the thyroid gland. Seaweed is important in this balance.

If you are taking blood thinning medication some caution is also necessary, as greens contain Vitamin K, which acts to thicken the blood, however some greens also contain more thinning agents and often there is the correct balance. Please speak with your medical practitioner about this.

Book:
The Choice - The Programme by Bernadette Bohan
Raw Juicing by Norman Walker
The Gerson Diet by Max Gerson M.D.

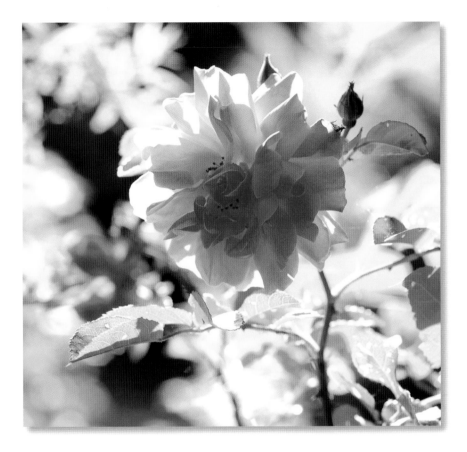

Karma,
Kindness, Knowledge

Karma

Karma is the total effect of a person's conduct during their existence. It is an ancient Eastern concept known by millions worldwide. It varies slightly among different traditions. It is the universal law of cause and effect. For each action there is an equal and opposite reaction.

In christian teachings it is the law of sin and death, and may be overcome by the love of God or the Holy Spirit. This is mercy.

Every thought and deed creates Karma, or in other words, consequences.

Once we become aware, and acknowledge recurrent unhealthy themes in our lives, we can take the opportunity to change these patterns. Conversely, we can use this law to create happiness – and reverse disease, even cancer!

> What you sow is what you reap.
> Mercy can wipe the slate clean.

Book:

The Tibetan Book of Living and Dying by Sogyal Rinpoche
The Law of Attraction by Esther and Gerry Hicks – The Teachings of Abraham
The Secret by Rhonda Byrne

Kindness

Kindness is a practice. Blessed are those who cultivate it – towards themselves and others. Kindness to oneself is not selfishness as is often felt.

One way of checking your own balance of giving and receiving is to do the Four Body Exercise by yourself or with another (see **Attention**).

Women, in particular, are "multi taskers" by nature, at least when younger, and are capable of giving a lot, often not knowing when the pendulum has swung toward over extending themselves. This is when resentment can stew and cause dis-ease, if not brought to the surface and acknowledged. Individual, as well as group support is generally needed for the balance to be corrected. Be patient with yourself if this is part of your make-up, and know that you have plenty of company! Learning to be kind to one's Self can be more difficult than being kind to others. It is often a point where women get stuck on their journey to wholeness, so finding your way to getting unstuck sometimes takes a leap of faith. Breast cancer is the motivator for many – the beginning of the next lap of Self discovery, and so the silver lining...

Book:
A Simple Path by Mother Theresa
CoDependent No More by Melody Beattie
Misunderstood – Mistreated by Ann Wilson- Schaeff
A Simple Abundance by Sarah Ban Breathnac

Knowledge

Knowledge is power. Try reading "Foods to Fight Cancer" by Professor Richard Beliveau and Dr. Denis Gingras, which contains a great explanation of cancer and how to prevent it naturally with foods. It also has some very interesting statistics.

It is the acting on the knowledge that really brings results, not just the knowing.

See **Websites**

Books:
Breast Health – The Wise Woman Way by Susan S. Weed
The Choice by Bernadette Bohan
Herbal Medicine, Healing and Cancer by Donald Yance Jr.
Cancer: Step Outside the Box by Ty M. Bolinger
Cancer-Free, Your Guide to Gentle, Non-toxic Healing by Bill Henderson

Notes

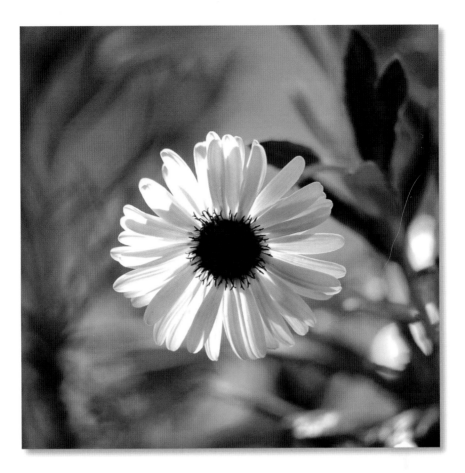

Laughter, Light,
Lineage, Listening, Longing,
Love, Lymph

Laughter

Laughter is still the best medicine! Find out what and who makes you laugh. Make it a priority. Movies do work. Check out Laughter on www.YouTube.com on a daily basis!

The immune system is boosted for up to 24 hours after a good laugh. It triggers endorphins which are the body's natural pain killers, as does exercise. It has been shown that the body cannot differentiate between fake and real laughter, so fake it if you have to, so you can feel better!

Laughter boosts your immune function by raising infection-fighting T-Cells, disease-fighting Gamma Interferon and B Cells. It lowers cortisol, the major stress hormone. Last but not least, it provides an opportunity for the release of emotions.

Book:

Laughter, The Best Medicine – The Healing Powers of Happiness, Humour and Joy by Robert Holden

Website:

www.YouTube.com (Laughter)

Google:

Laughter Yoga

Light

The light of day, regardless of sunshine, is important to our health and well-being to keep our hormones and biorhythms in balance. Our lifestyles have changed dramatically in recent years because of electric light. It has enabled us to have longer days and shorter nights, and to avoid the natural rhythm of the days and the seasons. This has been good for some things, but in the long run we may be paying the price by confusing our hormonal and immune systems. It is said that the sleep we get before midnight is the most important to health – "early to bed, early to rise, makes a man/woman healthy, wealthy and wise." Apparently it has been shown that even small lights left on at night will affect hormone levels negatively, and covering the eyes to make complete darkness is optimal. Ayurvedic medicine, the most ancient health system on Earth, tells us that it is best to begin to get ready for bed around 9pm, one reason being that cancer fighting and immune boosting cytokines are naturally secreted during these early hours of sleep. If you take note you will find that you naturally want to fall asleep at this time, but if you fight it and stay up, you will find it more difficult to sleep until later.

Humans used to live much closer to the Earth, in rhythm with the Sun and the Moon. With the advent of artificial light we have been able to manipulate and choose another way of life. Perhaps it has been an experiment, and as with any experiment there are results to be correlated. Maybe we need to take stock and make better choices to preserve integrity of the human body and psyche for ourselves as well as future generations.

Full spectrum lighting is an option for those who must be indoors much of the daylight hours. This will simulate sunlight, and has benefits for health and well being, especially those suffering from depression. This kind of lighting is probably best known for accelerating the growth of plants in winter.

Studies have shown that lack of Vitamin D (from sunlight) is an important factor in the occurrence of breast cancer. The effect of ELFs (electro low frequencies) from our modern technology based on electricity has also been shown to produce ill effects on our immune systems, and thus on apoptosis in the reduction of cancer cells.

It is unlikely that we will go back to all the "old ways", because electric lighting provides many benefits to our modern world (though some do want to experience this). However, considering that breast cancer (and prostate cancer in men) is an epidemic amongst women on this planet, there are some conscious choices that we can make to rectify this situation in relation to being in rhythm with the Earth, the Sun and the Moon. These choices would relieve stress, which some would say is the ultimate cause of any cancer.

Allowing our bodies and hearts to lead the way, rather than our heads, would be a good start to this revolution/revelation. This is not to say that we neglect our minds altogether – just that we come down a little nearer to the Earth and integrate all parts of us to embrace more wholeness. This in fact would be about bringing more of the feminine aspect to life, needed at this time in history to bring balance to the masculine aspect, which could be seen as running a little wild in years past! (The Celtic Tiger in Ireland?)

Remember that each of us holds both the masculine and feminine inside, regardless of our gender, and that each individual needs to integrate these to become whole.

In my opinion each woman who contracts breast cancer has an accelerated opportunity to find this balance, individually, collectively and globally, and thus find the light within herself. This of course applies to men too, if they should be one of the few diagnosed with this disease. (1%)

Books:
Light, the Future of Medicine by Jacob Lieberman
Sex, Lies and Menopause by T.S. Wylie with Julie Taguchi, M.D. and Bent Formby. Ph.D.
A Call to Power by Sharon McErlane

Lineage

Pay attention to your lineage to know yourself more fully. It cannot be denied, on any level.

The risk of breast cancer due to inherited faulty genes is 5%-10%; not as high as one is sometimes led to believe. However, if you have this risk you may want to pay extra attention to prevention and testing. Ask your doctor what he or she recommends. A second opinion could be worthwhile.

A strong family history of breast cancer could be:

> Two or more first degree relatives with breast cancer under the age of 50, or ovarian cancer at any age.

> A first degree relative with a known cancer gene.
> (You can be tested - ask your doctor for the BRCA 1 or 2.)

Some women choose to have a double mastectomy as breast cancer prevention if the risk is high, rather than have frequent mammograms and go through the anxiety of waiting for results each time. Another way of reducing this risk is through diet and lifestyle – making sure to eat the foods that fight cancer and keep your system alkaline as well as oxygenized.

See *Causes.*

Books:
Breast Cancer: Breast Health The Wise Woman Way by Susun S. Weed
How to Prevent and Treat Cancer with Natural Medicine by Dr. Michael Murray,
    Dr. Tim Birdsall, Dr. Joseph E. Pizzorno and Dr. Paul Reilly

Listening

As we listen to ourselves we can increase our capacity to listen to others.

This exchange is where much healing occurs. Time, money and confusion would be saved by allowing ourselves to listen more– and much illness could be avoided.

Remember to try that Four Body Exercise – again, and again.........!!!

Books:
Nonviolent Communication: A Language of Life by Marshall B. Rosenberg Ph.D.
The Silence of the Heart by Paul Ferrini

Google:
Nonviolent Communication

Longing

A longing lives inside each of us, buried in the recesses of our hearts. It is the longing for the Love that is inside and the source of that Love. We tend to get distracted and look for it outside, until we finally listen to the call that pulls (or pushes, as the case may be) us inside. At the core of every Spiritual Path is this Truth, with instructions to get there, with some deviation along the way perhaps! A pure intention with commitment is necessary to break through some old veils here. Look out for clues on this Treasure Hunt! The rewards are great.

A cancer diagnosis can be the silver lining to accelerate our pursuit of this Love inside ourselves.

Books:
Eat, Pray, Love by Elizabeth Gilbert
The Presence Process by Michael Brown

Love

Loving someone else is grand, but loving ourselves is grander, and ultimately more difficult, or none of us would need much healing, and disease would be negligible. If we could all find the Love that is inside ourselves and connected to our Source of Life perhaps it would be possible to eradicate cancer on this planet. So the challenge of breast cancer is to find this Love, inside our hearts, one woman at a time, until we reach the critical mass when the 100th monkey syndrome becomes apparent, and the Love Bug infects us all!

This requires us to live in the present moment – not the past, or the future. To fully embrace this we need to clear negative thoughts and emotions from our Being. How long this takes is unique to each of us. However, we are living at a time when this opportunity is accelerated, and miracles abound. The ancient Mayan people from South America who are very in tune with the cycles of the Earth, tell us that we are ending a dark age in 2012, so we are speedily clearing that which will not serve us in the coming brighter age.

Practice makes perfect, and if we commit ourselves, the Law of Attraction will give us all the opportunities that we need, in many forms, to succeed.

Books:
The Power of Now by Eckart Tolle
The Law of Attraction by Esther and Gerry Hicks: The Abraham Material
The Presence Process by Michael Brown
Love Without Conditions by Paul Ferrini

Lymph

The lymph system is a circulatory system of its own. It does not have a pump like the blood, and needs to be moved by our breath and the movement of our body, hence the importance of exercise. The lymph glands are part of our immune system and help to gobble up foreign matter, bacteria, viruses and abnormal cells. This system can be sluggish and get overloaded if it has to work too hard. Swollen glands are a sign of extra work needing to be done to eliminate particles of one type or another. Adequate water consumption helps to keep the lymph functioning well, along with adequate exercise.

One of the best ways to move the blood and lymph, (especially through your breasts) to detoxify, and strengthen your body and immune system is to invest in a small rebounder (not a trampoline, but similar) and bounce daily for 5 to 45 minutes, inside or out. Start with a short time and build it up, as feels good for you. It is rhythmic so becomes meditative. It can be done to music, or while watching TV, or outside in fresh air. There are degrees of manufacture, so it pays to do some research.

Remember to replenish your fluids – necessary to flush out the released toxins also.

The rebounder is a safe and good exercise post breast surgery. Speak with your doctor.

It is not necessary to jump off the base to get the amazing benefits of this form of exercise, said by NASA to be the most efficient exercise devised by man. It is the rhythm and reverberation of the bouncing which produces the effects.

A side effect of radiation and surgery for breast cancer can be a reduction in the flow through lymph glands under the arm, sometimes causing swelling and discomfort. This does not happen to everyone and there is no way of knowing who might be affected. If you do have symptoms a PhysioTherapist can be very helpful – even essential. Laser treatment is now available in many places for reducing this side effect. Literature and support groups are plentiful. Air travel can exacerbate symptoms, and you may want to prepare for this by wearing a stretch sleeve on your arm. You can be fitted for this, so please ask.

If you are prescribed exercises post surgery it is imperative that you do them, despite any discomfort. The consequences of not doing them are far more uncomfortable long term.

A good preventive measure for clearing toxicity from the breasts is based on kinesiology and is very simple. The trick is, like many other simple things, to do it!

It involves rubbing a sore point on the mid outside line of your thigh between your knee and your hip, while holding any congested part of the breast on that same side. Use whichever hands are easiest for you. See book below.

Book:
Your Breasts – What Every Woman Needs to Know – NOW! by Brian H. Butler

Notes

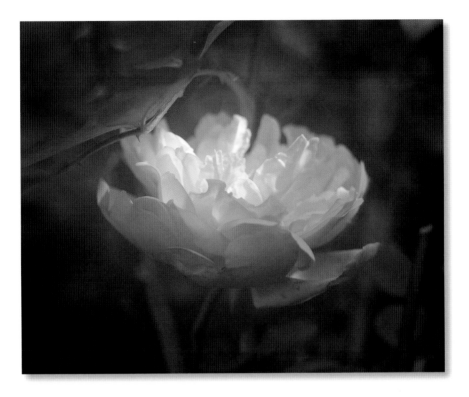

Meditation, Men,
Minerals, Mobile Phones,
Movement, Music

Meditation

Meditation is about the practice of listening and connecting to your inner self. Much has been written and taught about meditation from the spiritual standpoint. In more recent years research has proven the beneficial effects on the physical, mental and emotional level, as well as the spiritual. One trickles through to the other because of their connection.

Choose a method of meditation and/or a teacher that feels right for you. You can always change if you find something that does not resonate, though be careful not to miss a golden opportunity because of some discomfort.

Relaxing the body with some kind of movement and breathing can provide a good opening for reaching stillness within.

Meditation can be as simple as watching your breath with the sounds "SO HUM" or "HUM SA", which in actual fact may not be that simple to begin with! Practice makes perfect, and can take you to that place of love and stillness inside. Sacred sound and music, or a guided meditation CD or DVD are often helpful.

The added support of group energy can make a big difference.

Five minutes morning and evening is a good start, and can even become a wonderful addiction!

Books:
The Miracle of Mindfulness by Thich Nhat Hahn (also CD)
The Miracle of the Breath by Andy Caponigro (also CD)
Meditation by Sogyal Rinpoche

CD:
Mindfulness for Beginners by Jon Kabat Zinn

Google:
Vipassana

Men

The male population is of course greatly affected by the number of women dealing with breast cancer, as the female population is affected by the number of men dealing with prostate cancer. They are the same kind of tissue and as such are vulnerable in similar ways. Some of the solutions for prostate cancer are tied into the solution for breast cancer, and vice versa.

Women do not have prostate glands, but men have breasts, and about 1% of men do contract breast cancer. Men could catch early symptoms by doing a monthly breast self exam as women do, and report any irregularities to their physician.

Books:
The Men's Health Book by Dr. Mark Rowe
Men are from Mars and Women are from Venus by John Gray
A Call to Power: The Grandmothers Speak by Sharon McErlane

Minerals

Minerals are required for bodily function, including maintaining a healthy life force. There are seventy two trace minerals necessary for optimal functioning.

A lack of minerals equals a lack of life force. This is a common occurrence in our times because most soil has been depleted as well as overloaded with chemical fertilizers. These fertilizers are known to create an imbalance in the mineral content of the food, producing an acid medium which provides ground for cancer and other diseases. The importance of maintaining a correct supply of minerals in our bodies is paramount. This is one of the major reasons for eating organically, which means that the food has been grown in soil naturally fertilized, and without the addition of harmful pesticides. The bottom line is the health of the soil in which the food is grown as well as the freshness of the food one is eating.

During any stressful situation, including illness, minerals are needed in extra supply, through food, and sometimes supplementation.

Nettle tea has an abundance of minerals, as does fresh vegetable juice, sprouted seeds, wheatgrass, seaweed and soups.

Book:
Cancer: Cause and Cure by Percy Weston

Google:
Trace Minerals and Colloidal Minerals

Mobile (Cell) and Cordless Phones

Use protection from this vibration. ELFs (Electro Low Frequencies) and microwaves come from both your own phone, other peoples' phones and the transmitter towers (the masts positioned all around us – sometimes disguised as trees!). If you complain about lack of coverage, know that there will be more towers.

Some cell phone companies are apparently incorporating some protection in the manufacture of the phone, though this information is not given freely. Various methods of protection are now available. Look online, in your pharmacy and health food stores. Make enquiries for pendants, phone and computer buttons, crystals and various other personal, car and home devices.

Studies have shown that more than one of the same brand of button on your cell phone gives maximum protection.

Some people who use dowsing or kinesiology to affect change in energy will say that it is possible to alter the negative vibration of ELFs through thought and prayer.

It is advisable to become more conscious of your own mobile phone, where you keep it, how long you leave it on, and how often you use it.

Book:
ELFs by Robert Beckwith

Websites:
www.cancerfightingstrategies.com
www.dowsers.com

Google:
ELFs.

Movement

The lymph system helps to detoxify our bodies. It does not have a pump, as the blood does, and needs our breath and exercise of some kind to keep it moving.

Many people are using a gym these days to great advantage, with the added benefit of social connection. Care must be taken not to overdo here and cause undue stress and strain on the body.

Tai Chi and Qi Gong are gentle and powerful.

Hatha Yoga is excellent, and does not have to be strenuous. Restorative yoga is good when you are recovering from any illness or surgery and are more vulnerable. There are good books and teachers available. Check with your health practitioner post surgery or during illness.

Walking is perhaps the best, most natural and simplest movement. Research shows that the health benefits of even a little walking are enormous. The added element of fresh air, sunshine and nature make it the perfect package.

Swimming and rebounding are other excellent ways to move your lymph. It is said by NASA that rebounding is the most efficient exercise devised by man. Five minutes is equal to a thirty minute walk. Astronauts combat the unnatural effects of being in space by bouncing on this "mini trampoline." Calcium is restored to the bones, as well as other health benefits.

Remember that if you are unable to do any of the above exercise, it is possible to move some parts of your body quite adequately while lying, sitting or standing. Even resting your feet on a rebounder while someone else bounces (and this can be done without lifting one's feet) brings excellent results!

Please see *Exercise*.

Books:
The Health Benefits of the Rebounder by Albert Carter
Kundalini Yoga by Shakta Kaur Khalsa

Music

Our body is a symphony, made up of sounds. It constantly needs tuning. Choose sound and music that harmonise your soul to keep healthy. Sing, sound and listen! Treat yourself to a portable CD Player and a set of good headphones – you will be amazed how the music permeates your body, mind and spirit.

Books:

Return to Harmony – Creating Harmony and Balance through the Frequencies of Sound by Nicole Lavoie

Music and Sound in the Healing Arts by John Beaulieu, N.D.

The Healing Power of Sound: Recovery from Life Threatening Illness using Sound, Voice and Music by Mitchell L.Gaynor, M.D.

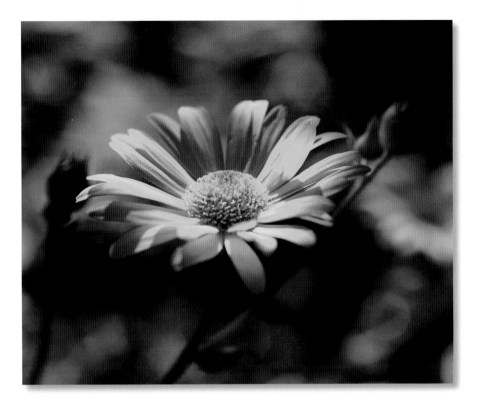

No, Nutrition

No

Catch yourself when you are saying YES when you really mean NO!!!

A good rule for changing this pattern, if you do it, is to train yourself to take a deep breath when asked to do something, whether appealing or not, and then say you will think about it, before you actually commit. This gives you time to get to your most truthful answer, which believe it or not, will take better care of every one, including you, which may not have been the case when saying yes.

It can take some time to get over feeling selfish and guilty with this one, but it's worth a try. The rewards can be life saving.

Books:
CoDependent No More by Melodie Beattie
Co-Dependence: Misunderstood – Mistreated by Ann Wilson-Schaeff

Nutrition

Nutrition can be one of the most confusing subjects, as there are so many different points of view. It can also be one of the most difficult aspects of our lives to change. Sharing food is also a social ritual and we tend to like to fit in with others rather than be different. Consequently, if we are serious about changing our lifestyle habits we sometimes need to spend less time with some people and more with those in alignment with what we are striving for, or spend more time alone.

One of the most widespread and unknown reasons for the cause of cancer is the lack of nitrilosides (otherwise known as Laetrile or Vitamin B17), found in many green grasses, plants, grains, seeds and fruits, especially stoned fruits such as apricots.

Eat slowly. Remember to chew your food well –
the digestive process begins in the mouth with your saliva.

A health practitioner knowledgeable in nutrition is necessary to guide you with changes in your diet, especially if you have a diagnosis of cancer. Be aware that there are different options here, such as a dietician, a naturopathic doctor or a certified complementary nutritionist. Each practitioner will work from their own unique perspective.

Exploring the ancient system of Ayurveda from India can be very illuminating, even if only to discover your particular "dosha" of Vata, Pita or Kapha. This can be found by doing a short questionaire available in books or on the web. Knowing your blood type and perhaps following some of the nutritional suggestions for your type, could be very helpful, as well as giving some guidelines and reasons for living a more healthy and harmonious life according to your type.

Please see **Digestion, Juicing, Minerals, Organic, Oils, pH Balance, Food Combining, Supplements** and **Treasures**.

Books:

Healing with Nutritional Therapy by Patricia Quinn

The Body Ecology Diet by Donna Gates and Linda Schatz

The Gerson Therapy: The Amazing Nutritional Program for Cancer and Other Illnesses by Charlotte Gerson and Morton Walker, D.P.M.

The MacroBiotic Approach to Cancer by Michio Kushi

Perfect Health: The Complete Mind Body Guide by Deepak Chopra M.D.

Live Right for Your Type by Peter J. D'Adamo N.D. with Catherine Whitney

Foods to Fight Cancer - Essential Foods to Help Prevent Cancer By Professor Richard Beliveau and Dr Denis Gingras

Prescription for Nutritional Healing by James F. Balch, M.D. and Phyllis A. Balch, C.N.C.

The China Study by T. Colin Campbell Ph.D. and Thomas M. Campbell II

Cancer by Matthias Rath, M.D.

Prannie Rhatigan's ***Irish Seaweed Kitchen***

Websites:

www.bodyecology.com

www.dadamo.com

www.dr-rath-foundation.org

www.hippocratesinst.org

Notes

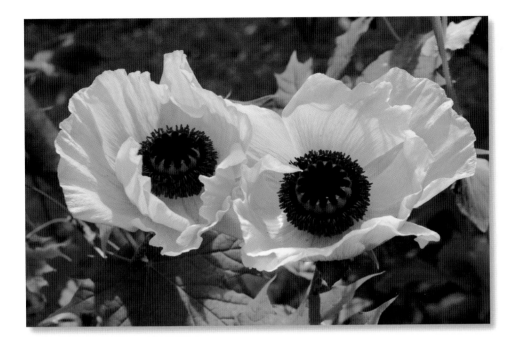

Oils,
Oncology, Organic,
Oxygen

Oils

Oils are an extremely important component of good health.

They deliver essential nutrients such as fat soluble vitamins and essential fatty acids to our cells. It is said that the greatest nutritional deficiency currently affecting North American and European countries is the low intake of polyunsaturated fatty acids of the Omega-3 variety. People who eat an unhealthy diet tend to get more Omega-6 than they realise because it is the primary oil added to most processed foodstuffs, which creates an imbalance.

There are several different types of oil, some of which are more beneficial than others. Some are even anti-health, - that is, cause disease and death.

Monounsaturated fats such as fish oils, olive and flax oil have a protective effect on our health. Saturated fats such as animal fats and hydrogenated oils (trans fats) contribute to our health problems, especially when they are heated, e.g. all fried foods. Refining of fats and oils has virtually eliminated essential fatty acids from the food chain.

Dr. Johanna Budwig discovered in her research of fats and oils related to health that the one common denominator for all cancer cells was the mal-absorption of fats and oils. One of her theories is that oil holds a large amount of sun energy, which is what we humans thrive on. Flax oil becomes water soluble and free flowing when bound to protein compounds of sulphuric content such as cottage cheese, or quark. The cheese loses its negative dairy effect when combined with flax oil. There are alternatives for those with a severe dairy allergy.

Statistics show that Greece has a lower incidence of breast cancer than most countries, which is possibly explained by their consumption of large amounts of olive oil daily.

Heating cold pressed virgin olive oil produces free radicals, so this is best kept for raw consumption such as salads, pouring over vegetables, and as a replacement for butter.

Olive oil does not have an abundance of essential fatty acids, but does have other health enhancing properties, such as cholesterol reduction and blood thinning. Too much consumption of one type of oil can cause a deficiency in another type, necessary for our health. eg. over consumption of olive oil (Omega-3) can lead to deficiency of Omega-6, in certain diets.

Organic unrefined coconut oil or ghee (clarified butter) and grapeseed oil are the healthiest oils to use for sautéing. This is because they remain stable when heated.

Fat digestion is of course of the utmost importance if you are going to increase your intake of any oils. Digestive enzymes with a high lipase content are helpful here. If these oils are a new addition to your diet it is advisable to begin with small amounts to allow your body to adjust.

There isn't much point in spending money on good food if you are not digesting properly and producing toxins that will make your body work harder, or overload it perhaps, leading to discomfort, fatigue and consequently disease.

To be kind to yourself and your liver, buy your oils organically grown, cold pressed, unrefined and in dark glass bottles. Your liver does not have the ability to process refined and chemically extracted oils. Store your oils in the refrigerator, except for olive oil, which can keep up to three years away from light. Some oil can be stored in the freezer if you buy in a large quantity.

Certain fish have an abundance of Omega-3 oils and are very easily digested by most people. However fish oil, though beneficial, is not a mandatory essential oil.

There are other choices if you are vegetarian. Caution is advised around the source of the fish, as pollutants are in some waters more than others. Salmon, one of the top fish for healthy oils, is mostly farmed these days and contains only half the oil, approximately, of wild salmon caught in the ocean. This is dependent on the food they ingest.

Most oils in supplement form have a very short shelf life, so read labels and dates when buying, and exercise caution.

Emulsifying oils, by blending or mixing, enhances the absorption process greatly. This allows the oil to bypass the liver and go directly to where the oil is needed in the body, which can make a vast difference. Salad dressings give us the opportunity to emulsify.

Books:
Fats that Heal: Fats that Kill by Udo Erasmus Ph.D.
The Body Ecology Diet by Donna Gates and Linda Schatz
Foods to Fight Cancer by Professor Richard Beliveau and Dr. Denis Gingras
True Health against Arteriosclerosis, Heart Infarction and Cancer
   by Dr. Johanna Budwig

Oncology

There are many people alive today because of modern day oncology, (the study and treatment of tumours - Oxford Dictionary) which is ever experimenting and changing. Side effects of radiation and chemotherapy drugs can be difficult, with nausea, loss of hair and digestive disturbance being the most common. That people accept this is a testimony to their wish to live. There is also evidence to show that oncology is not always life affirming. It can kill cancer cells but also other healthy cells, as well as severely damaging the immune system, which is needed to keep check on cancer cells.

However there are ways to counteract the negative effects, one of which is keeping a positive attitude. Research is showing us better ways, and each person who has made this choice has contributed to our learning.

Each doctor who is willing to help in the ways that they know, must be commended for the risks they take to save live, and find a more compassionate way.

A German clinic has found a way to test cancer cells for specific chemotherapy, rather than giving it generally, with great success. They also give substances for the immune system prior to treatment, as well as colour therapy via light. Some clinics in America and other countries are now exploring this route.

Treatment for cancer often depends on what one's consciousness evokes, one's level of fear and perhaps one's curiosity and education on the subject. Availability of treatment and financial resources are a major consideration, as well as one's desire to live and become more conscious.

A note on supplementation and oncology:

This subject is under much scrutiny and there is controversy about the taking of supplements while undergoing treatment. For instance, it is said that antioxidants can counteract the positive effects of chemotherapy. However, there are other studies to show that taking them is better than not. This is an individual choice. It is something to be discussed with your specialist and may depend on the type of drug that is prescribed.

Books:

The Key Model by Dr. Sean Collins, B.A.(Psych)D.C.H. and Rhoda Draper, B.A (Psych) Dip.C.H.

How to Prevent and Treat Cancer with Natural Medicine by Dr. Michael Murray, Dr. Tim Birdsall, Dr. Joseph E. Pizzorno, Dr. Paul Reilly

Organic

Organic means that food is grown consciously in relation to the earth and humankind - for health, not against, unlike chemical pesticides and fertilizers, though some kinds are less harmful than others and are useful. Buy organic, grow organic and eat organic as much as possible. It is essential for good health, especially if one is recovering from an illness. One of the major reasons for eating organically is the imbalance that chemicals (fertilisers and pesticides) produce in minerals, thus making a body environment conducive to cancer and other diseases. The other is that we do not need to ingest any more foreign substances into our bodies, which are already compromised on many other levels. If there is a diagnosis of cancer all the energy in our system needs to be available for detoxifying what is already there and for facing this challenge.

Book:
Cancer: Cause and Cure by Percy Weston

Oxygen

In 1931 Otto Warburg was awarded the Nobel Prize for discovering that cancer cells survive well without oxygen, and conversely do not survive well in the presence of high levels of oxygen. As a result of this he recommended a variety of treatments based on oxygenating the tissues.

Oxygen is paramount to healthy cells, hence the value of exercise and of deep breathing daily. However oxygen cannot reach cells that are acidic, so this is another confirmation of the importance of alkalising our systems, by means of hydration, nutrition, stress reduction, emotional release and geopathic stress correction. An Italian M.D. Dr. Tullio Simoncini has discovered an inexpensive way of alkalising tumours with sodium bicarbonate, though controversial.

A hyperbaric oxygen tank is an option. Google.
Oxygen drops are also available, as well as portable Oxygen Cannisters, at a reasonable cost.

Websites:
www.phmiracle.com
www.alkalizeforhealth.net
www.simoncini.com

Notes

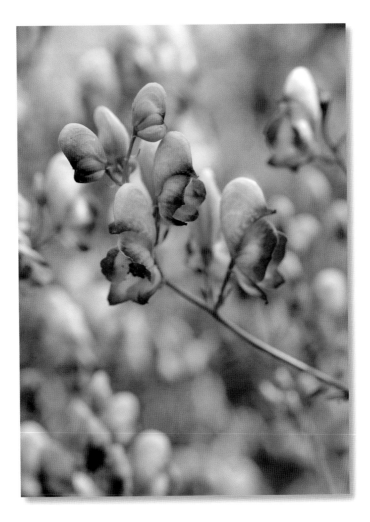

Pain, Patterns,
pH Balance, Phytochemicals, Prayer,
Procrastination, Psychotherapy

Pain

Pain can be reduced by hypnosis, relaxation techniques, guided meditation, loving touch, energy healing, acupuncture, a Tens Unit, as well as by various over and under the counter medications. Reduction of pain is directly related to endorphins – substances which are released in our bodies, triggered by pleasant experiences as well as healthy exercise. From an energetic perspective, pain manifests if there is not enough energy in a part of the body, as in hip and leg pain because one is operating too much in the head, or from the spiritual body.

Pain on any level is directly related to all the other levels (or bodies) of our Being. For instance physical pain will have an emotional component, which in turn is related to a mental pattern. All of these are connected to our Spiritual Body – or disconnected, as the case may be.

Use of medication, drugs, alcohol, food, cigarettes and any addiction can suppress the real cause of the pain, and thus stunt our growth and awareness, and keep the cycle repeating rather than changing it. Another way of approaching this is to explore the reason for our addictions, (we all have them) which will inevitably uncover a memory that will come with emotional pain and a need to change if we are to become more responsible. This can explain why we are resistant to releasing our addictions. Support and professional help is very necessary for a smoother transition, and there are now ways to make this graceful and relatively painless. Those who have gone before us have inspired us to evolve processes of seeking help.

Books:
The Presence Process by Michael Brown
Tapping Your Way To Health by Roger Callahan, Ph.D. with Richard Turbo

Google:
Thought Field Therapy

Website:
www.emofree.com

Patterns

We are somewhat like computers and can be programmed with various viruses, (or patterns) which need to be eliminated. We pick a lot of them up before the age of seven through our energy system from those with whom we spend most time - parents, teachers, relatives, friends, spiritual mentors – and TV and movies!

Patterns can manifest positively and negatively. How to judge? Those that stop the flow of our Life Force and our connection to our selves are negative, and those that open that connection to our selves are positive.

Part of our life's work is to become aware of our patterns and transmute them, so as to know who we are and why we are here. If this were easy we would have been enlightened long ago. The difficulty is that the patterns are stored in our subconscious minds and are not accessible by our conscious minds until we are ready to explore this, one level at a time. In truth, our subconscious is always a mirror reflecting back to us from our lives and those around us, and when we recognize this, every moment becomes an opportunity for awareness and growth. This is expertly explained in the book below by Michael Brown.

Psychotherapy, Hypnotherapy, NeuroLinguistic Programming, Kinesiology, Energy/Body Work, Clairvoyance and Regression Therapy, are some of the ways through which we can become more conscious, and give ourselves the opportunity to change our patterns for the better.

Help with this is sometimes found as information from other levels of consciousness. This is sometimes known as "channeling".

Google:
Esther and Gerry Hicks – The Abraham Material

Books:
The Presence Process by Michael Brown
The Journey by Brandon Bays

pH Balance

The pH measures the acid/alkaline levels of our body fluids, such as saliva, urine and blood.

The pH of the blood is very important to the health of our cells, and ought to be between 7.35 and 7.45. Our food, air, hydration, thoughts, emotions, breathing and stress all have an influence. We have a natural buffering system which works to balance this mechanism when we are healthy. However, over time our diet and lifestyle can overwork this system and cause an imbalance. We can then become more acidic and vulnerable to disease, including cancer.

We tend to become more acid than alkaline with a heavy protein diet, especially meat. Coffee, sugar, trans(formed) fats, processed foods, alcohol, lack of minerals, insufficient chewing and incomplete digestion are other culprits. Refined vinegar is another offender and is in many foods. Read the labels. However, unpasteurised cider vinegar that contains the mother culture in a dark bottle is alkaline forming. The use of this as a regular drink is very much an individual question because of how it works. Testing for its compatibility with your body, especially if you have a cancer diagnosis, is advisable. Bacteria, viruses and fungi thrive in acidic blood, so it benefits us to keep more alkaline most of the time with leafy green vegetables, sprouts, some grains and some fruits. Cancer cells do not live in an alkaline medium. Acidic blood is lacking oxygen, which is also conducive to cancerous activity.

Some of the top alkaline foods are Lemons, Watermelon (eaten alone) Daikon Radish, Seaweeds, Seasalt and Ginger.

Google:
Alkaline forming foods – detailed list.

Exercise sometimes produces lactic acid and toxins are released, making our blood temporarily acidic. However, breathing deeply and rapidly while exercising, and afterwards, gives our bodies an opportunity to release carbon dioxide which will revert your blood to an alkaline state. If more lactic acid is produced than the body can handle then an acidic state will continue. Exercise coaches know the solution to this, as do some nutritionists. Extra water intake will help to balance this syndrome also and detoxify the acidic waste.

106

Books:

The pH Miracle by Robert O. Young Ph.D. and Shelley Redford Young
The Body Ecology Diet by Donna Gates and Linda Schatz
Killing your Cancer without Killing Yourself by Allen S. Chips D.C.H, Ph.D
The Macrobiotic Approach to Cancer by Michio Kushi and Edward Esko

Websites:

www.thepHMiracle.com
www.alkalizeforhealth.net
www.naturalnews.com

Phytochemicals

There are more than a thousand phytochemicals in plants which regulate our hormonal balance and protect us from diseases. They are contained in almost all foods except those which are refined.

The ones we are most familiar with are:

> Lycopene (tomatoes)
> Isoflavones (soy)
> Flavanoids (fruits and vegetables)
> Carotenoids (yellow fruits and vegetables)
> Polyphenols (green tea and grapes)
> Indoles (cabbage and brussel sprouts)
> Sulforaphanes (broccoli and brussel sprouts)
> (Increases enzymes which detoxify cancer forming chemicals.)
> Allylsulfides (onions, leeks and garlic)
> Capsaicin (hot peppers)
> (Protects DNA from carcinogens.)
> Terpenes (citrus and cherries)
> Saponins (beans)
> Proanthocyanidans (cranberries)
> (They prevent the adhesion of pathogens to our cell walls.)

Most of these phytochemicals have antioxidant properties; in other words they protect cells from oxidative damage, so help us reduce the risk of developing cancer.

In relation to breast cancer, Isoflavones are the most important because they are phytoestrogens, which take up the natural space for oestrogen, thus not allowing the more harmful oestrogens room to break in.

There is some concern about Genistein, one of the two phytoestrogens in soya. In some studies it has been shown that it can negate the effectiveness of the drug Aromatase (Letronole), sometimes given in the treatment of breast cancer to reduce the level of oestrogens.

Please see **Hormones**.

Books:
The China Syndrome by T. Colin Campbell
Sex, Lies, and Menopause by T. S. Wiley with Julie Taguchi M.D.,
 and Bent Formley, Ph.D.

Prayer

Prayer is about intention and feeling from the heart. It is about faith in knowing that what you ask for is already done - on some level. It is a science combined with faith and feeling.

One can potentially make one's life a prayer.

Thought, Sound, Movement and Visualisation can all help with this.

Different cultures and spiritual paths provide formulas to guide us in our prayers, though everyone can create their own, straight from the heart, beginning with gratitude for what we already have. Repetition and practice are often required, human beings that we are, though once can suffice. Group prayer intensifies the invocation. Much benefit can be gained from saying prayers on an ongoing basis, as a blessing or as protection.

Each word, sound and thought creates a specific vibration that reverberates through our bodies and out into the Universe, with the potential to come back to us, boomerang-like. It is important to be open to receiving the answer to our prayer. This is where many of us have difficulty, and need to explore our resistance to fully receiving, or believing that we will receive. Perhaps this could be our priority prayer – to clear the obstacles to receiving, belief or lack of, and receptivity!

Clarity of intention accelerates the miracle of an answered prayer. Exploring intention through verbalising, writing or meditating can be very helpful in finding clarity. Miracles abound by the minute…

Here's a sample suggestion for praying:

> Breathe deeply as you connect with your heart:
> Clarify your Intention:
> Feel the feeling:

> Connect with your source of spiritual sustenance such as God, Great Spirit, Angels, Guides, Mother Earth or whatever feels right to you. Give thanks for their Presence and assistance. This can be done out loud if desired. If none of this resonates with you just connect with your breath, upon which your Life Force travels.

> Express your gratitude and feeling verbally in the present tense e.g. "I am grateful for all that I have, for the gift of Life, for my body which is a vehicle for Love, and for my health in this moment. May I be a blessing for all those with whom I am connected." (i.e. everyone everywhere!)

Move to music, knowing that each movement danced from your heart sends out a wave of Peace, Love, Joy, Health or whatever it is you are invoking.

Make any sounds that want to be expressed -high, low, soft or loud or if you have a chant you enjoy saying or singing this could be a good time for that, unless you would like to begin with it.

End with a time of silence, however long or short. Notice if you feel different. Make an effort to keep the mainstream of your thoughts positive, while acknowledging the not so positive ones.

Books:
The Law of Attraction by Esther and Gerry Hicks – The Abraham Material.
Benedictus – A Book of Blessings by John O'Donoghue
Peace is every Step by Thich Nat Hahn

Website:
www.howardwills.org

Procrastination

Procrastination can cost you a lot, even your life. If you write down what you know you are procrastinating about - what you are putting on the long finger - you can take a good look and see what you **will** do. Then you can choose to take some action, or not, very clearly.

Help from a friend, therapist or coach is very valuable here for accountability (See **Four Body Exercise** under **Attention**).

Psychotherapy

Seeking out the help of a psychotherapist/counsellor sooner rather than later is a very good move. One does not need to be sick or in pain to begin any kind of therapy, though most of us need the prompting of either or both. There are many forms of psychotherapy. Most therapists will use a combination of techniques incorporated with their own unique style. Ask your health practitioner or friend for a referral.

Books:
New People Making by Virginia Satir
The Continuum Concept by Jean Liedloff
The Presence Process by Michael Brown
The Miracle of the Breath by Andy Caponigro

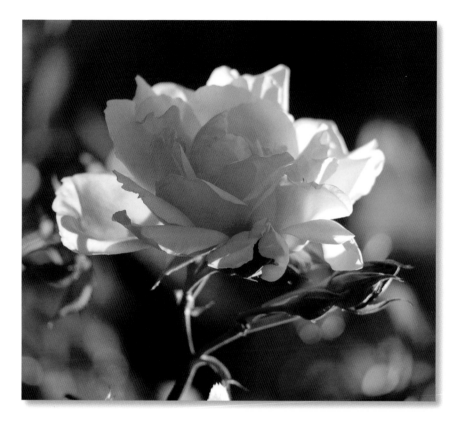

Qi, Questions, Quiet

Qi/Chi

There are other words for Qi/Chi, such as Life Force and Prana. Every health tradition has a name for it. This is connected to the breath and its path along the meridians of the body, which fuel each cell and organ. This "substance" is ultimately responsible for the integrity of our energy system and our entire health. Acupuncture is one system that uses the flow, or blockage of flow of energy to diagnose and treat various conditions. Awareness of this has not generally been taught in conventional medical school, though monitoring of the pulse, blood pressure, temperature, respirations, reflexes and other responses are indications sometimes equivalent.

Many devices measure these flows and their blockages both in conventional and alternative medicine. Computer technology has advanced our knowledge in this respect. Mammography, thermography and ultrasound are some examples of showing us where Life Force or Chi can be lacking or in a healthy flow.

Biofeedback technology is often used in alternative medicine to detect imbalances in someone's energy field, and consequently help to elicit change. Disease is where the flow of energy, whatever name you give it, is altered in some way from its original blueprint. There are many ways this can happen.

Learn Qi Gong, Tai Chi or Yoga. Walk, breathe, go out in nature. Know that every movement creates Chi and with intention has powerful effects. Watch your thoughts, your company and your environment. Eat good food. Drink pure water. Be conscious about the type of cosmetics that you use. Check your degree of geopathic stress.

Be aware that everything has a vibration. Live your life from this perspective, and if you want to raise your vibration to its highest potential surround yourself with that which will support this endeavour. (eg. Meditation, Exercise, Nutrition, Spiritual Healing and Psychotherapy)

Relapse is often part of the journey! See **Addiction**.

Books:
Wuji Gong by Grand Master Wei Zhong Foo
Da Dao Chan Gong by Grand Master Wei Zhong Foo
Healing Light of The Tao: Foundational Practices to Awaken Chi Energy by Mantak Chia
Energy Exercises by John Chitty and Mary Lousie Mueller
The Power to Heal: A Clear, Concise and Comprehensive Guide to Energy Healing by Roberto Pellegrino-Estrich

Questions

Please ask them.

Write a list of questions for yourself, your doctor, other health care practitioners, and for your buddy/coach.

Make friends with your fear and ask anyway.

Books:
An Alternative Medicine Definitive Guide to Cancer by W. John Diamond M.D.,
    W. Lee Cowden M.D. with Burt Goldenberg
Cancer – Step Outside the Box by Ty M. Bolinger
Cancer Free by Bill Henderson
Sex, Lies, and Menopause by T.S. Wiley

Websites:
www.cancerstrategies.com
www.healingcancernaturally.com

Quiet

Quiet can be difficult to find these days, both inside and out. Time seems to have speeded up, and indeed it actually has. The Earth has gone from a speed of 12 Hz to 16 Hz in the past years! This results in our minds racing a little faster too, as we try to catch up with ourselves. Technology and noise, whether it be music or machines and computers, bombard us every week, if not every day, with new information which our brains attempt to assimilate. A feeling of being overwhelmed is common for men, women and children. When we need quiet more than ever, it often escapes us, unless we can manage to go away to some sanctuary, which can go a long way toward bringing balance to our lives. Many of us have a constant longing for this kind of quiet. It can be found in our own environment if we make the choice to create it. Making a vow of silence for yourself for any length of time will give you surprising sanctuary in your own body and mind if you have the courage and willingness to undertake this.

Notes

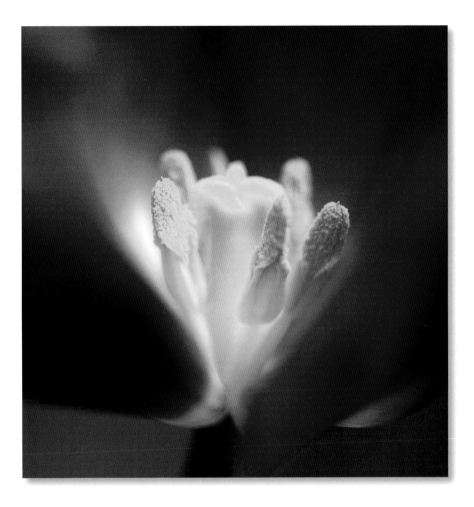

Radiation,
Receiving, Relationships,
Rest, Rhythms

Radiation

See *oncology* and *chemotherapy*.

Receiving

We feel loved when we are received. The open heart receives unconditionally. We need to do this with ourselves also.

Rejection is the cause of much pain – rejection of ourselves as much as from another. The other is merely a reminder and reflection of what we do to ourselves. If we practice receiving another we practice receiving ourselves. If we love another we are feeling the depth of our own love. Expectations are responsible for much disappointment and disharmony. Letting them go is not always easy but a goal to be strived for perhaps?

Books:
Silence of the Heart by Paul Ferrini
Unconditional Love by Paul Ferrini

Relationships

Good relationships can bring much comfort through love, companionship and common goals. These are seldom easy all the time because they are ground for growth on all levels. Some would say that intimate relationship is a spiritual path, requiring the commitment and practice that any path of this sort demands. Each two people come together for their own reasons, based on the Law of Attraction, their intention and their subconscious patterns.

Relationships can be the cause of much conflict, resentment and despair - some of the precursors of cancer. However, it is all opportunity for Self examination and growth toward wholeness, though the wounding that can occur is very real and can take time and support to heal. The rewards can be great for those who dig deep and face the challenges.

Communication is the first and highest choice to resolve issues. Professional help is a wise step, and can make the difference between ending or keeping a relationship.

Sometimes ending it is the most appropriate action, though it can be difficult. This does not mean that the love is lost - just that the framework for that love needs to change for both people to expand and fulfill their needs.

Blame never works. It is more useful to note what we see outside ourselves and then to look inside, using the issues as an opportunity for self reflection, and moving forward – perhaps away from a victim stance.

Lived well, an intimate relationship, based on honest communication, willingness, heart felt love and commitment can bring much joy through sharing life.

Books:
Journey of the Heart by John Wellwood
The Presence Process by Michael Brown
Intimate Communion by David Deida

Rest

Most women need more "down time" than they are getting. This lack creates imbalance and diminished Life Force/Chi.

This is about changing a pattern, even a collective pattern for women, (an archetype) and can be more challenging than one might think. Go deep to find your resistance to Self nourishment on this level. Do seek help if you need encouragement.

Books:
Archetypes by Carolyn Myss
CoDependent No More by Melody Beattie
Co-Dependence: Misunderstood – Mistreated by Ann Wilson Schaef
Meditations For Women Who Do Too Much by Ann Wilson Schaef

Rhythms

The Sun, Moon, Stars and the Earth have rhythms which affect our bodies, the oceans, the animals, the plants and all of life, creating harmony if adhered to. However, most of humanity seems to have decided that it is not necessary to pay attention to these rhythms, much to its detriment. Each organ of the body resonates in rhythm and sound with the others, and has certain requirements to keep this connection harmonious. Much of modern life disregards this and then wonders why ill health prevails.

Some simple corrections can be made with the use of light and dark, using the principles of sound to harmonise situations and the body. We can learn to listen to our bodies, as well as practicing the art of Qi Gong. The awareness that everything is Energy and has its own frequency is helpful because then we can know when we are not resonating in harmony with our surroundings, which can include people. Noticing the behaviour of animals can be a good guide for us, as they live well in tune with nature.

Book:
Cellular Awakening by Barbara Wren

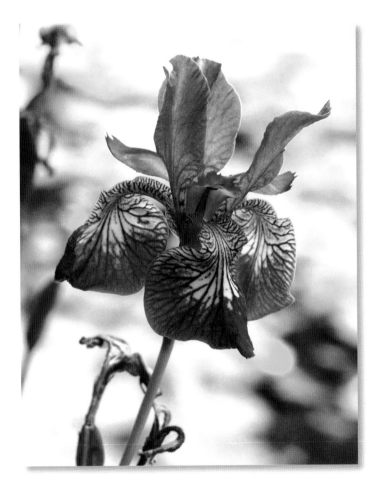

Sexuality, Sleep, Sound,
Spiritual Healing, Sprouting, Stages,
Statistics, Stress, Subconscious,
Sunshine, Surgery, Supplements

Sexuality

Sexuality is probably the most misunderstood subject on planet Earth by the majority of people, causing untold misery and suffering, when it could in fact cause a pandemic of spiritual bliss, if there were more education and less prejudice in this arena. However this, no doubt, will evolve like everything else.

It is not commonly known that Kundalini, which is spiritual energy, lies dormant at the base of the spine, and when activated, as can happen with sexual activity and certain exercises and breathing, will connect one (either alone or in partnership) with one's source of Love, God, Spirit or whatever one likes to call it, which is what we are all looking for anyway. However it is necessary to cleanse old thoughts, patterns and habits to be able to get to this, and some training and education is helpful. This often comes under the name of Tantra, which is a path of Yoga, embracing all aspects of our Being. This is becoming more available now all over the world, whereas before it was kept more secret, as people were not ready to change. It is a positive sign of our times that this is so.

Women in particular know at a cellular level what they need and hold sexually but are often not conscious enough to express this and so the unconscious manifests as illness, particularly in the breasts or reproductive system. As each woman comes to know and heal her own wounds, as well as discover the power of her own sexuality, illness of this type will decrease and eventually be unknown, one would hope.

Professional help is necessary most of the time for most people, as these wounds run deep and wide.

Books:
The Return of Desire by Gina Ogden Ph.D.
Healing Love through the Tao: Cultivating Female Sexuality by Mantak Chia and
 Maneewan Chia
Taoist Secrets of Love: Cultivating Male Sexuality by Mantik Chia
I Remember Union by Flo Aeveia Magdalena

Google:
Kundalini Yoga
Tantra/Tantric Yoga
David Deida

Sleep

Lack of sleep causes all sorts of problems such as a compromised immune system, a rattled nervous system and impaired memory – to name a few. In short, sleep is one of the most healing things around, so it makes sense to pay attention if you are not getting it.

Ayurvedic medicine, in particular, suggests heading for bed around 9pm. The early hours of sleep are when the most cytokines are secreted. These substances naturally boost the immune system, and fight cancer cells. The hours between 10pm and 2am are said to be the time when our body repairs and detoxifies itself.

Seek professional help if over the counter herbs, homeopathy or relaxation therapies are not working.

Your favourite music with headphones can be very soothing.

It can be really helpful to get things "off your chest' and out of your mind, and perhaps subconscious also, by talking with a friend, housemate, spouse or sometimes a therapist.

Try to end your day with a sense of completion. This can be an excellent time to write in your journal. Take note of the good things that happened in the day, not just the things that have been troubling.

See breathing exercise under **Breath**.

A word here on Serotonin, an important neuro-transmitter for sleep, anxiety, depression and mood control, sometimes known as the happy neuro-transmitter.

When certain foods which contain Tryptophan (one of the eight essential amino acids not manufactured in the body) are properly digested they are converted into serotonin, necessary for calming and mood balance, as well as influencing peristaltic action in the gut. Some of the foods high in Tryptophan are turkey, brown rice, oats, fish, eggs, mung beans, sunflower seeds, cottage cheese, pineapple, bananas, spinach and sardines.

Sound

Sounds can be soothing or irritating to our system. Your energy, gut or heart will let you know which is which. It is a good idea to pay attention and to avoid the irritating ones as much as possible. Even if you are not known as a musician or singer you can experiment with your voice and with any instrument to express yourself.

Beat a drum. Strum a guitar. Ring a bell. Sound a quartz crystal bowl, or a Tibetan singing bowl to change and raise the frequency of your vibration.

Join like-minded people and create a sound healing circle.

Books:
The Healing Power of Sound: Recovery from Life-Threatening Illness using Sound, Voice and Music by Mitchell L. Gaynor M.D.
Music and Sound in the Healing Arts by John Beaulieu N.D.
Return to Harmony by Nicole Lavoie

Spiritual Healing

If our Spirit is fully connected to our source of life, breath and energy, and we are living from that place with honesty and commitment, then there is no room for illness. However this is what Earth School is about, and it ain't that easy!

Any person who helps us with this endeavour to connect more to ourselves and our Source, whatever one may call it, is giving us spiritual healing.

Some people have trained, or have the gift of bringing more awareness through Light or Energy, without words, and can open us to more of ourselves, and thus eventually to more health. Energy healers are worth seeking out.

Books:
The Power to Heal: A Clear, Concise and Comprehensive Guide to Energy Healing by Robert Ester Pellegrino
Hands of Light by Barbara Brennan

Websites:
www.FriendsoftheCasa.info
www.HowardWills.org

Sprouting

Raw, live sprouts contain much nutrition and precious enzymes. They can be bought in health food stores as well as regular supermarkets now, or you can grow your own. Please buy organic. They are very easy and inexpensive to grow, giving you cheap food.

Some possibilities are alfalfa, wheatgrass, sunflower, peas, lentils and mung beans. If you are a beginner in sprouting, like anything new, it requires instructions, focus and persistence until it becomes second nature and a habit. In this instance it is well worth it, and can be life saving. It is also fun!

Books:
Sprouts: The Miracle Food by Steve Meyerowitz
Health Building: The Conscious Art of Living Well by Dr. Randolph Stone, D.O, D.C.

Google:
Primal Seeds Sprouting
YouTube Sprouting

Stages

There are four stages of breast cancer generally recognized by the medical profession. Palliative care is given in the fourth stage in conventional medicine, as well as ever increasing chemotherapy medications to prolong life, though each case is individual and there are always exceptions. Alternative medicine does seem to have more success with fourth stage cancer through nutrition, psychotherapy, affirmations and spiritual/energy healing, etc. often in conjunction with conventional methods.

Website:
www.breastcancer.org

Statistics

Breast cancer is the second leading cause of death in women today, lung cancer being the first. More than a million people in the world will be told that they have breast cancer this year. One in four women with cancer have breast cancer and 50% of these women live in developed countries. Despite new development in technology and drugs, the rate of survival still leaves a lot to be desired. Ireland has the highest survival rate for cancer in general in Europe.

Deaths from cancer worldwide are projected to continue rising with an estimated twelve million deaths in 2030. More than 70% of cancer deaths occur in low and middle income countries. This is presumably because of lack of education and access to treatment.

It seems that prevention would counteract much of this loss of life as well as high cost of treatment, and the distress caused by illness and loss of work, in whatever capacity.

Stress

In a German study cancer cells have been totally annihilated by reducing stress and inducing relaxation on a consistent basis. This is possibly due to the change in the pH balance of the blood from an acid to an alkaline state.

Stress is anything that puts an unhealthy pressure on the body. We each respond in our own unique way to these pressures, depending on who we are, how we think and feel, how we view the world and our current state of mental health. What fills one person with fear may invigorate the next one.

Stress can be brought on by psychological upset, fatigue, surgery, noise, resentments – the list is endless. Our nutritional needs soar the more pressure we encounter.

Stress puts a huge demand on our adrenal glands which respond by releasing cortisol, adrenalin and noradrenalin. We can continually release these substances when under constant stress, rather than when they may be needed in a particular situation. If they are not used up with physical exertion, they lodge in our systems and cause many problems, not least of which is diminished immune function.

Exercise not only disperses the harmful substances, but releases serotonin, the happy neuro transmitter. This seems a rather pleasant way to counteract the effects of stress and insomnia (and constipation!) if one is well enough and makes the time. (see **Sleep** and **Constipation**) It has been shown that even minimal movement makes a significant difference to our wellbeing.

Deep relaxation and meditation have also been proven to counteract the effects of stress. Fifteen or twenty minutes morning and evening are optimal. The benefits are enormous. You can begin by using a relaxation audio. Some practitioners will help you create your own personal CD. The yogic path provides relaxation through movement, breathing, sound and meditation, so a yoga class is one way of incorporating preventive medicine in your daily or weekly routine.

The most important aspect of reducing stress is to examine our lives on all levels and see what we want to change to bring about good health and balance in this fast paced world in which we live.

See **Attention** for **Four Body Exercise**.

Bodywork of any description is a wonderful antidote to stress. It can be expensive. Students need bodies to work on! Sometimes those close to you are willing to rub heads, feet and/or hands. When there is a diagnosis of cancer speaking with your health care practitioner before getting massage is advisable. Contrary to some beliefs massage can be quite advantageous, but there are sometimes contraindications to certain methods in specific situations. There are now massage therapists trained for people with a cancer diagnosis.

Books:
Kundalini Yoga by Shakti Kaur Khalsa
The Power of Now by Eckart Tolle – also Audio
Letting Everything Become Your Teacher by Jon Kabat-Zinn
The Miracle of the Breath by Andy Caponigro
Meditation by Sogyal Rinpoche

Subconscious

Ultimately the subconscious leads the way. Check in with it frequently and work to harmonise it with your conscious mind. Seek professional help if you can, and are willing. This can be scary territory, and the ego is not always willing! However, integration of the conscious mind is necessary to become whole, however one does it.

Dreams are a good way of showing us the subconscious mind. They are not always remembered, but with intention to do so before sleep, this can be improved upon. Deficiency of the B Vitamins, especially B6, can prevent our dream recall.

You are your own best interpreter, but help can enhance your perspective, shedding light on some aspect of your life which needs attention.

Books:
The Presence Process by Michael Brown
The Miracle of The Breath by Andy Caponigro
Healing Trauma: Restoring the Wisdom of the Body by Peter A. Levine (also audio)
The Journey by Brandon Bays

Sunshine

The Roman Historian, Pliny, wrote "Of all the remedies the sun is the greatest". It increases both red and white blood cells and therefore improves the immune system. The ability of white blood cells to eat up cancer cells is very much enhanced. The sun balances our hormones, improves liver function, and normalises circulation. Muscle tone is increased. Mood is elevated.

The heat of the sun can also be stressful if too much is taken in, especially if one is ill. The rays of the sun are very powerful and need to be treated with respect. Today the holes in the ozone layer around the Earth do not provide enough protection from the harmful rays. It is said that fifteen minutes daily in the sun with the body half exposed four months of the year is enough to absorb your daily quota of Vitamin D. Your time in the sun should be before 10am and after 3pm approximately, depending on the latitude and time of year. There is debate on this subject. Others will say that just exposing your face and hands five minutes daily will be sufficient.

Many sources now show that the lack of Vitamin D can encourage the growth of breast cancer cells, and that if women had enough of it there would be much less of this disease.

The oil in our skin contains Vitamin D2 and when the sun hits this there is a chemical reaction that makes Vitamin D3, which is what we need. Some time needs to elapse between sun exposure and skin washing - so be aware of being too clean!

Full spectrum lighting can be an important adjunct for those who live in the northern hemisphere and do not get enough sunshine in the winter months (or summer months!) due to their lifestyle. This lighting is available in ecological/green stores.

Vitamin D supplementation is sometimes necessary, as one in two people are apparently deficient. A blood test is available to find out levels of this vitamin. Other methods of a more alternative nature include kinesiology, biofeedback devices and clairvoyance.

Google: Full spectrum lighting

Books:
Sex, Lies, and Menopause by T.S. Wiley with Julie Taguchi, M.D., and Bent Formby, Ph.D.
Light: Medicine of the Future by Jacob Lieberman
Flax Oil as a True Aid against Arthritis, Hearth Infarction, Cancer and Other Diseases by Dr. Johanna Budwig

Surgery

Surgery is sometimes miraculous. Much dedication, learning, skill and risk taking is required by a good surgeon, and there are many. As in any profession, there are various levels.

There are many grateful people walking around post surgical procedure.

It is now quite well accepted, thanks to Peggy Huddleston, that we can programme ourselves while under the influence of anaesthesia. Many anaesthesiologists are very willing to co-operate with this.

Book:
Prepare yourself for Surgery by Peggy Huddleston

Supplements

Much controversy surrounds this subject.

Ideally one tests daily for supplements, or at least weekly, if one is taking them. It is useful to learn some way of testing ourselves, such as with the pendulum or with kinesiology. Find a good knowledgeable nutritionist and see what he/she has to say, and then use your own wisdom with this. Your local health food store will have information on practitioners.

A good basic multi-vitamin covers a multitude. A food based one is good, but not always sufficient in case of deficiency.

Co-creation is a responsible way to go. When you agree on a plan it is advisable to follow it consistently. This makes all the difference.

See *Treasures* and *Heather's Top Tips for Optimal Health* after Z

Books:
Supplements Exposed: The Truth They Don't Want You To Know About Vitamins, Minerals And Their Effect On Your Health by Brian Clement
The Vita-Nutrient Solution by Dr. Robert Atkins
How to Prevent and Treat Cancer with Natural Medicine by Drs. Michael Murray, Tim Birdsall, Joseph E. Pizzorno and Paul Reilly

Notes

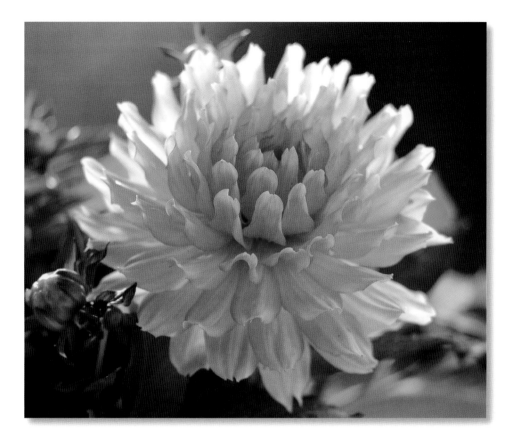

Teeth, Tests, Thymus
Touch, Trapped, Trauma,
Treasures, Types

Teeth

It has been shown in Germany that the state of our teeth directly affects organs in the rest of our bodies to quite a degree, so it is important to make good dental care a part of our health regime – and not necessarily the last part. The tongue, gums and mouth reflect the state of our health, as well as affecting our health, and need our attention daily.

Some people will advocate removing all teeth with crowns and root canals for reversing disease of all kinds, especially breast cancer. This does not mean that everyone needs to follow this advice. Careful consideration is advised, as well as some kind of testing for each individual.

Book:
The Cure for All Cancers by Hulda Clark, Ph.D., N.D.

DVD:
Cancer Conquest by Burton Goldberg

Tests

There have never been so many tests available before, and more appear every day.

There is one at least, for every level of consciousness, and most parts of us.

The advent of the computer has accelerated our ability for testing. Biofeedback technology is now being used both by private practitioners and hospitals, e.g. the Vega, Eclosion and Life Machines, as well as the BEST, QXCI and SCIO.

Google practitioners in your area, though some of these therapies are as effective done long distance, where you can stay in the comfort of your own home.

A common test for breast cancer (and ovarian cancer) in conventional medicine is a blood test called the Ca 125. This is called a cancer marker. There are others.

There is also a test to ascertain if a woman is carrying the gene for breast cancer BCRA 1 and 2.

Two other tissue tests done mostly when the cancer diagnosis is aggressive are the Ki-67 and the uPA+PAI-1. They are both helpful in determining the best treatment for complete recovery. There are more tests of one kind or another being researched on a daily basis. Ask a physician, or breast cancer specialist for the most up to date testing.

In Ireland, Dublin City University (DCU) is conducting a trial with women for a possible breast cancer marker in blood serum. This is based on the enzyme Seprase, and could be an exciting new potential for very early detection of breast cancer. A positive test could avoid the necessity for a biopsy.

Orthodox Medicine also offers Mammograms, Ultra Sound, Magnetic Resonance Imaging, (MRI), and Biopsy. Mammograms and Biopsies are more invasive than the others, but often prove very useful, despite some side effects and recent bad press. These techniques are being examined and often improved on a daily basis. Thermography is sometimes offered in a conventional setting, but more often in an alternative center. This is a system of utilizing heat senstivity in the body with photography and can detect abnormalities in the breast long before cancer manifests, but accuracy depends on good preparation. Following directions is imperative here, and then this methodology can be extremely helpful, and perhaps worth paying for from your own pocket in conjunction with other opinions.

A new genomic test (genes) very recently has shown that each individual case of breast cancer can be tested to ascertain the correct type of chemotherapy for the most efficient result. Research is being finalised for marketing and treatment in the future. Some clinics in Germany and USA have already been treating people based on this. **www.burtongoldberg.com**

Another trial study is being conducted between Irish and American hospitals to measure a woman's need for chemotherapy after surgery, (tissue is necessary) based on something called oncogenes. It has been discovered that it is not always necessary for complete recovery. **www.mytreatmentdecision.com**

The AMAS test measures the Anti Malignant Antibody in Serum and appears to be quite accurate in detecting the level of cancer cells anywhere in the body, especially in the early stages. It does not detect tumours above 4 cm in diameter. This test can be good reassurance after treatment of breast cancer to keep a check on reoccurrence, and allay fears. The downside is that it is only available in one lab in America, and it requires blood to be mailed overnight in dry ice. It is stated that it has a 95 to 97% success rate, and has been known to detect cancer cells one to nineteen months before clinical testing. For some reason very few people know about this test, including doctors, even though it has been around for over 20 years, and is covered by health insurance. Some added research seems to be required to make this test respected by more people.

Medical Clairvoyance can be used in conjunction with orthodox and alternative medicine, and in some clinics is part of the plan.

Ideally, testing is done in more than one method for optimum accuracy and security, as no one method is 100% reliable. False positives and negatives are apparent in all forms.

One of the most reliable ways of testing is the Breast Self Exam done regularly. More breast cancers are found in this way than any other.

Google:
AMAS Test

Website:
www.youtube.com/selfbreastexam

Thymus

The thymus gland rules our immune system. It sits above our heart (and energetically is part of it) and behind the breast bone. It is much influenced by our feelings. Happy feelings produce a strong immune system and prolonged, worried or shocked feelings can produce a weak immune system.

Research has shown that cancer can manifest after a very stressful time in one's life if feelings are not dealt with appropriately, and enough support is not available. This also depends on an individual's chemistry, personality and life history.

Tapping the chest bone and sounding Ahhh...simultaneously is a good way to boost the thymus gland.

Book:
The Miracle of the Breath by Andy Caponigro

Touch

Given with love, and no agenda other than to give comfort to the person receiving, touch is one of the most healing events in life. It brings relaxation, which allows self healing. It relieves fear. It opens the meridians of the body to allow more Life Force to flow and deepens the breath.

It sometimes produces profound realisations and connection to one's Source of Energy – God, Great Spirit – Angels and Spirit Guides.

Friends, relatives and partners may all be willing to participate in giving and/or receiving touch – a foot rub or head massage for even ten minutes can make a world of difference.

Look for a practitioner in your local health food store, or holistic magazine. Ask for a referral.

Book:
The Polarity Experience by Richard Gordon

Trapped

Explore ways that you may feel "trapped" in any part of your life. Work to free yourself. This is often an inner struggle projected outward. Seek the inner first, and take responsibility for your current situation and how it was created. Find professional help, either individual or in seminar/workshop form.

Acceptance (see **Acceptance**) may also be the lesson needed in some situations.

Book:
Leaving Abuse Behind by Sarah Daniel

Trauma

Trauma is often stored in our cell memory, blocking energy, which can manifest as disease and imbalance on any and all levels. This trauma can have been so injurious that survival requires that it is hidden in the subconscious until such time as one is willing to bring the trauma to light. Sometimes it is pain, a life challenge, or illness (eg. cancer) that pushes us to explore the whys, and to get help with this journey. At this time in history there is more awareness and there are more tools available for efficient and compassionate healing. Everyone needs them at some stage in their lives – the sooner the better, though there is such a thing as Divine Timing.

It has been discovered in Germany that all cancer has a trauma registered in some part of the brain, and if this is accessed and healed, then the cancer heals. This theory has not been very well supported, despite a very high success rate.

Google:
Dr. Ryke Geerd Hamer

Books:
Healing Trauma: Restoring the Wisdom of the Body by Peter A. Levine (also audio)
The Miracle of the Breath by Andy Caponigro. (also a CD)
The Presence Process - A Healing Journey into Present Moment by Michael Brown
The Journey by Brandon Bays

Website:
www.emofree.com

Treasures

Please note that there are different needs for cancer prevention and for a cancer diagnosis.

Wheatgrass	Barleygrass
Sprouted Seeds and Legumes	Raw Fruits and Vegetables.
Raw Juices	Spirulina/Blue Green Algae
Flax Oil and Cottage Cheese	Flax Meal
Flax Oil	Olive Oil
Nuts and Seeds	Bee Pollen
Bee Propolis	Garlic
Ginger	Onions
Turmeric and Black Pepper	Asian Mushrooms/Beta Glucans
Cruciferous Vegetables	Sea Vegetables
Berries/Ellagic Acid	Digestive Enzymes
Probiotics	Aloe Vera
Nettle Tea or Juice	Green Tea
Apples (raw and stewed)	Pure Water
Raw Dark Chocolate	Niacin
Flower Remedies	

Types

Go to **www.breastcancer.org**

A less common form of breast cancer called Triple Negative has had a bad prognosis in the past, but conventionally certain new chemotherapy drugs are having very good success rate, so there can be less fear with this diagnosis. Alternative methods can also be explored, either as support or as a separate journey. Supervision from a health provider experienced in this particular type would be preferable, though the choice is always up to the individual.

Notes

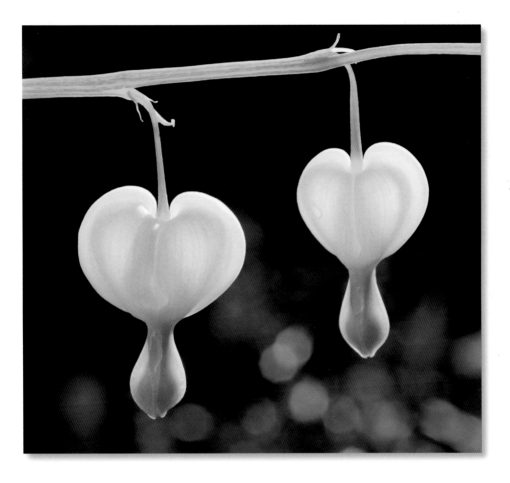

Unawareness,
Unique

Unawareness

We are all unaware of some things, probably even the most aware of us. This is why a team or group approach helps learning – we learn from each other.

Many of us get impatient with the level of our own awareness. We must remember that there is joy in the journey – and wisdom gained.

Hindsight is 20/20 vision they say.

Self acceptance is the key and staying in the present moment brings awareness. Our male-oriented culture does not encourage this, producing much stress and anxiety, which leads to disconnection from our Soul, and thus disease.

We need the balance of masculine and feminine for our very survival, and the survival of the Planet. This applies to all of us, male and female.

Book:
A Call to Power: The Grandmothers Speak by Sharon McErlane

Unique

Honour your uniqueness. Generalisation is useful only up to a point. Be sure to ask yourself if what you are doing is resonating with you on all levels. If not, ask yourself what needs to change.

What's good for the goose is **<u>not</u>** always good for the gander.

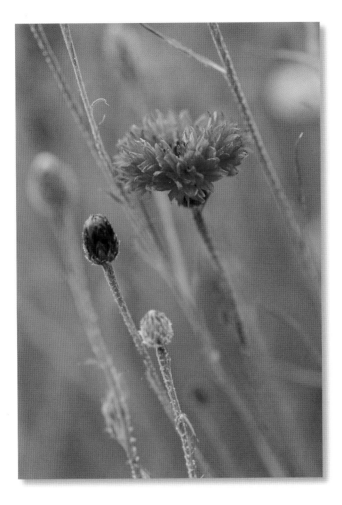

Vacation, Vibration,
Visualisation, Vitamin D,
Vulnerability

Vacation

It seems that two weeks in succession is necessary to relax and rejuvenate. Three is optimal.

Vacation for one person is not the same as for another. Make sure you get what you need.

Finances are necessary for taking this kind of time off, and not everyone can see where to find the necessary resources. Getting clear about your intention, writing it down and talking about it to friends and relatives could bring you closer to your dream, which does not have to be elaborate.

Sunshine is imperative, wherever and whenever you get it. Our cells thrive on it, and need it for health. We do get it through foods that absorb and store sunlight, but our skin also needs it directly for hormone health, bone health, Vitamin D and Calcium absorption, nerve health and relaxation.

It is said that the safest, most healing rays of the sun are before 10am and after 3pm, avoiding the most harmful rays, allowing for difference in latitude, and time of year.

Vibration

Everything in creation vibrates to its own sound and wavelength, including human beings. There is a blueprint for perfection contained in everything, and sometimes deviations occur.

Any illness is an opportunity to come back to our perfect blueprint, and live our life from there.

This blueprint, while in human form, requires maintenance and servicing, as with all other vehicles!

Immortality may be possible, but many of us have contracts for a particular life path for a certain length of time. We elect certain experiences for our learning, and when we have completed this we are ready to leave. There are many ways to do this. Cancer is one of them. Sometimes we can change the contract in mid stream by desire, willingness and by grace through prayer. Sometimes not.

We may choose again, and continue on a new life path.

Much can be learned through the dying process, and healing at death can be profound, for the one experiencing it, as well as for those closest.

Book:
The Tibetan Book of Living and Dying by Sogyal Rinpoche

Visualisation

This can be a large part of your ticket to complete healing.

See Attitude and Affirmation – the law of energy following thought combined with visualisation and conscious intent has the power to change all the molecules in our cells. Conventional, as well as Alternative Medicine, is giving more and more credence to this, and so it is possible that we will be seeing visualization and positive affirmations more widely used as a routine part of cancer treatment in the near future.

Add a healthy diet, detoxification, and pure water and good health is a strong possibility!

There are many stories to confirm this.

Books:
Creative Visualisation by Shakti Gawain
You Can Heal Your Life by Louise Hay

DVD:
Cancer Visualisation: Return to Wholeness with Deepak Chopra M.D.,
    David Simon, M.D. and Dr. Stephanie Simonton

Audio CD:
Cancer Recovery with Louise Hay

Google:
Youtube visualisationbreastcancer
Youtube Louise Hay

Vitamin D

Studies have shown that breast cancer could be much reduced if women were getting enough Vitamin D, either through sunlight or supplementation. Many other diseases are linked to this lack also.

Vitamin D is unique in that it is a vitamin, but it functions as a hormone. It is fat soluble and so needs to be consumed with some kind of fat to be absorbed, if it is taken orally. It can also be taken sublingually so as to bypass the digestive system. The natural way to receive it is through sunlight. It is difficult to get enough from food, especially with any digestive or liver disorder. It can be taken in supplement form as Vitamin D3.

It is recommended to take 400 to 800 iu (international units) of Vitamin D3 to prevent illness. A food based calcium supplement or food equivalent needs to be taken with this to prevent toxicity if you are not getting exposure of at least your hands and face to sunlight (without sunscreen) for at least fifteen minutes a day three times a week, or equivalent. Different advice will be given on this as more exploration is done on the subject, so do your own research and use your discretion. A blood test can easily measure your level of Vitamin D. It is a fat soluble vitamin so it is stored in the liver - consequently too much can also be a problem, so some caution is needed in taking this as a supplement.

The immune system vitality is directly related to the concentration of Vitamin D in the body. It also has a direct effect on our calcium metabolism, and magnesium is an even more important factor in this equation. If the body lacks magnesium, neither calcium nor Vitamin D will be utilized optimally. Please seek out a practitioner knowledgeable in this subject. Some of these facts are not commonly known, though are recently coming more into the public eye. A naturopathic doctor or medical herbalist would perhaps be good avenues for advice. People at risk of Vitamin D deficiency are those who are indoors much of the time, shift workers and those who consume a lot of carbonated drinks. Excess animal protein and calcium intake has been shown to inhibit benefits of some Vitamin D.

Dark complexioned people are also at risk because their skin is a natural protection from long hours of strong sunlight, and so does not absorb as much as light skin. This does not serve them well if they are not getting an extra dose of strong sunlight.

Let us not dismiss the fact that UV radiation from the sun is carcinogenic. This fact needs to be well respected. It is responsible for a large number of skin cancers annually. This may be due mainly to the thinning of the ozone layer which leaves us more vulnerable to these rays. Each person needs to find their own healthy balance for optimal health.

People who have had certain types of gastric bypass surgery will not absorb Vitamin D through food because this vitamin is synthesized in the part of the upper small intestine which may have been bypassed. This also applies to those with any digestive absorption problems, as well as those on anti-convulsant medications. In these cases sunlight would be even more important.

The medical profession in general will say that Vitamin D can be absorbed through a sunscreen up to a factor of approximately 80, which most people do not need. Conflicting advice can also be found.

One needs to be aware that whatever is put on the skin becomes food for the body, so your choice of sunscreen needs to be considered. There are some safer than others that will still do the job, though they may be a little more expensive, and sometimes not as easily applied. However a good search will find you the right product for your needs.

Alternating between several different good sunscreens is perhaps a prudent choice.

The main foods that contain Vitamin D are sockeye salmon, tuna, mackerel, eggs, dark green leafy vegetables as well as sprouted alfalfa and sunflower seeds.

Vulnerability

Honour your vulnerability, sometimes hidden. We often mask that fragile part very well from ourselves and others. Being vulnerable can be a scary thing, especially because of its power.

Illness exposes our weakness, as well as our strength, and can give us the opportunity for integration. To have this met with compassion is a great gift.

Books:
The Miracle of the Breath by Andy Caponigro (CD also)
The Presence Process by Michael Brown

Notes

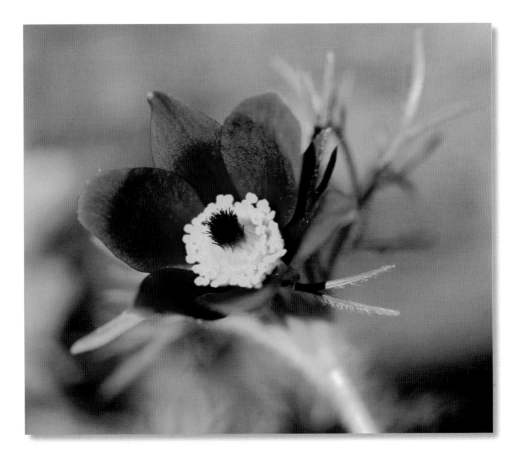

Water, Websites, Willingness

Water

Who would ever have thought that we would be spending such a sizeable amount of our pay cheques on good water? And in plastic bottles? As we drink pure water we throw plastic into the earth. Recycling saves us somewhat. The side effect of the convenience of some cheaper plastics can be cancer producing – as we drink our "pure" water!!!

Our bodies are 70% water and need to be replenished continually with good water – minus chlorine, lead, aluminium, flouride, pesticides and other chemicals.

Regular detoxing of heavy metals is advised for optimal health. It has been said that they are very carcinogenic.

We pay a price for material greed and the manufacture of substances without thought of future consequences. Native Americans ask us to consider seven generations ahead – a wise and kind request.

A jug filter for water is simple, though not optimal. Flouride (still in Irish tap water) is not eliminated with this method.

More efficient filters can be fitted to the sink and also for the whole house. Reverse Osmosis is one of the ways of doing this. In all cases it is imperative to clean or change the filters when needed, or before. Otherwise there isn't much use in bothering with any of it.

Healthy water manifests in certain molecular structures naturally for health and is found in less and less places now. Healing waters are shown to have this structure, but we can also create this for ourselves with intention, blessing, symbols, light, magnets, alkalizing and ionizing. There are also glass and other products being made now to return water to its original healthy structure. Drinking water left in a cobalt blue glass bottle in the sunlight for one hour will give you an extra boost. Writing any positive intention on this bottle (or any container) will send this vibration to the water and thus to your body and psyche - eg. Love, Respect, Compassion, Peace, Gratitude. Mineral water is often sold in these blue glass bottles, or they can be purchased.

Some people say that dehydration is the primary cause of cancer due to the fact that our bodies become extremely acidic and thus deoxygenated – the perfect ground for cancer. So perhaps paying attention to how much water and what type we are drinking would be a first step to health. The calcium, magnesium and potassium balance are also of utmost importance. (See BarbaraWren's book on Cellular Awakening.) Dehydration is when inadequate water reaches our cells. The amount of water that you require will depend on your diet, mineral intake, state of health, climate, and if you are also drinking caffeine in any form, or alcohol, which are diuretic and so dehydrate your body. Mental activity, stress and exercise require extra fluids. Sipping is known to be more efficient than gulping!

In Morocco the women who work in the fields will bring Argon oil with them to take, rather than copious amounts of water, which is heavy to carry. Apparently the oil will lessen the need for water and keep correct hydration, due to its holding qualities, so this signals the importance of ingesting correct oils in keeping our hydration balance, though this is not a generally known fact and may need more investigation. Some will say that oils keep the skin lubricated so that evaporation of water does not occur so quickly.

Good salt, such as Celtic Sea Salt or Himalayan Salt, also have this effect of keeping the fluids in the body.

Water has enormous curative powers, as long as it is pure.

It is possible to have your own water tested locally, or by mail online. It would be optimal to get the most comprehensive available.

Google:
Water Filtration, Water Ionization, Reverse Osmosis

Books:
Water: The Ultimate Cure by Steve Meyerowitz
Your Body's Many Cries for Water by F. Batmanghelidj
The Healing Power of Water by Masaru Emoto
Cellular Awakening by Barbara Wren

Websites

www.irishcancersociety.ie
www.arccancersupport.ie
www.macmillan.org.uk
www.pennybrohncancercare.org

www.canceradvice.co.uk
www.breastcancer.org
www.mytreatmentdecision.com
www.breastcancersupport.org
www.curenaturalicancro.com
www.cancerfightingstrategies.com
www.burtongoldberg.com
www.beating-cancer-gently.com
www.thewolfeclinic.com
www.enzymestuff.com
www.cancerx.org
www.cancure.org
www.alkalizeforhealth.net
www.healingcancernaturally.com
www.alternative-cancercare.com
www.colourtherapyhealing.com
www.hippocratesinst.org
www.louisehay.com
www.dowsers.com
www.vitalaffirmations.com
www.yogalaughter.com
www.howardwills.org
www.friendsofthecasa.org

Willingness

Stubborness seems to be inherent within the human condition. Ask yourself where you are willing and unwilling to change, and be realistic. Seek help if and when you are willing!

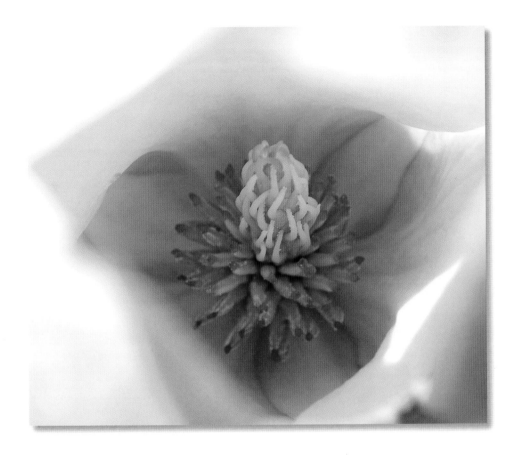

X (Avoid), X-ray

X (Avoid)

Let's face it, some people have stronger constitutions than others, and can get away with all sorts of things. Perhaps their livers function well to detoxify their systems. However, continually going against nature will catch up with them eventually, perhaps even in future generations.

General Rules:

For optimal health and cancer prevention please avoid the following as much as possible:

Sugars, and other acidic foods
Drinking too much alcohol
Being indoors too much without air exchange
Suppressing emotions
Cooking food in aluminium
Grilled and charcoaled foods
Food additives
Overeating
Chemical cosmetics
Flourescent lighting

Smoking
Breathing noxious fumes
Negative thinking
Eating trans fats, cooked meats
    in excess, rancid oils
Chips and crisps
Impure water
X-rays
Household chemicals

X-rays

X-rays have a certain amount of radiation which is cancer producing in high enough accumulated doses. The benefits may outweigh this risk and technology has improved, but do take stock of this fact, and perhaps look for alternatives. MRIs, PET scans and CAT scans all produce a certain amount of radiation.

Ultra-sound is less invasive, as is Thermography. Some of the more alternative would be Kinesiology, Dowsing, BioFeedback Technology and Medical Clairvoyance.

A Trans Atlantic Flight is equal to three or four X-rays. Taking some anti-oxidants and/or immune enhancing products for a few days before and after your flight can counteract this. Homeopathy and Flower Remedies can also be very effective, as are copious amounts of water.

Book: *Cancer Free* by Bill Hendersen

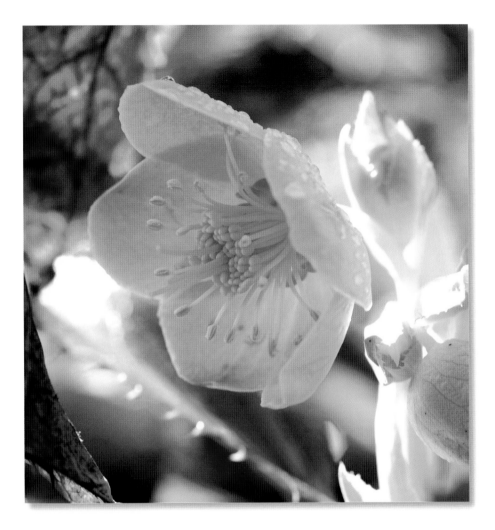

You, Yoga

You

There are many fun ways to get to know ourselves.

We can use Meditation, Movement, Self Reflection, Journaling, Psychotherapy, Drama, Creative Expression, Channeled Readings, Self help Books, Tapes and DVDs.

Know your Ayurvedic constitution.
Explore your Astrological chart.
Find out your Numerology, and your number in the Enneagram system.
Explore your Archetype.
Know your Blood Type.
Check your Iridology.
Log your Dreams.

Books:

Perfect Health by Deepak Chopra
Archetypes by Carolyn Myss
The Complete Idiot's Guide To The Power Of The Enneagram by Herb Pearce, M.Ed., with Karen K. Breese, PhD.
The Life You Were Born To Live: A Guide To Finding Your Life Purpose by Dan Millman
Linda Goodman's Sun Signs by Linda Goodman
Live Right For Your Type by Dr. Peter D'Adamo

Audio:

Magical Body, Magical Mind by Deepak Chopra

Yoga

Yoga is a scientifically-proven, non denominational spiritual path addressing all levels of human evolution. There are many derivations available now, with excellent teachers. Some names you may find are as follows:

Hatha, Kundalini, Iyengar, Ashtanga, Bhakti, Vinyasa

Books:

Kundalini Yoga by Shakti Kaur Khalsa
Yoga For Your Type: An Ayurvedic Approach by Dr. David Frawley and Sandra Summerfiel Kozak M.S.

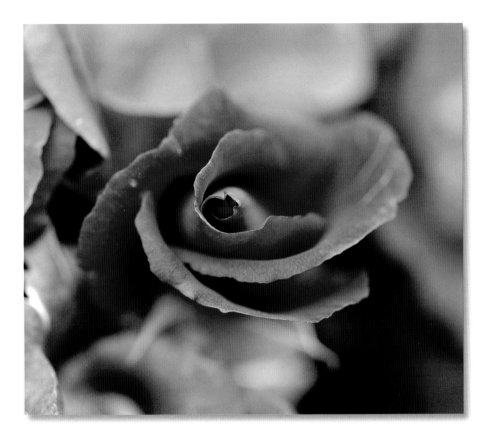

Zapping

Zapping

Zapping is a relatively new phrase in the world of health, originating with Dr. Rife, the creator of the Rife Machine. Dr. Rife gave each micro organism and disease a number, and his machine changes the vibration so that particular organism or disease cannot live in the altered state – quite ingenious and painless.

You can make your own "zapper" as directed by Dr. Hulda Clark, or it can be bought ready made.

The Rife Machine can be a separate entity or included in another device. It is always recommended to use this in conjunction with other healing methods, and under supervision. There has been some controversy about Dr. Rife's methods and zapping, but nevertheless there are many success stories. Testing with kinesiology or dowsing could evaluate whether the Rife machine could be useful in each individual case, and if there were any contraindications.

Books:
The Cure for All Cancers by Hulda Clark, Ph.D. N.D.

Website:
www.huldaclark.com

Google:
Rife Machine or Dr. Rife

Heather's Top Tips For Optimal Health

Breathe.......I mean really breathe..... a little time in fresh air for extra intake of oxygen, and a dose of sunshine if possible. Practice alternate nostril breathing once daily at least.

Move/Exercise............these two, as well as Laughter, are probably the best medicine and counteract many weaknesses.

Watch funny movies.

Smile - whether genuine or not, this releases good hormones.

Drink enough Pure Water, and filter your shower water too!

Use Sound ....Sing and Chant....... Listen to Music. Make your own Music.

Meditate, even for 5 minutes a day. Create Space and Silence for your Self.

Eat Organically. Read labels on everything!

Eat a Balanced Diet, with the emphasis on maintaining an Alkaline pH.

Eat sufficient Raw Foods to ingest valuable Enzymes.

Chew your food well – you are what you digest.

Ensure that you have regular bowel movements.

Detox periodically, and check for Parasites.

Release negative thoughts and emotions, while affirming positive thoughts daily. Learn a tapping technique such as EFT (Emotional Freedom Technique) to help with this.

Check your levels of Resistance, Resentment, Conflict and Despair regularly – by yourself, and with another.

Check your home environment - exchange household and cosmetic chemicals for less harmful products.

Protect yourself from Electromagnetic and Geopathic Stress.

Use Full Spectrum Lighting in some locations in your home and office. Avoid fluorescent lighting.

Get enough sleep, whatever that is for you.

Learn to listen well to others.

Learn to listen to your body, as well as your head.

Talk less, but speak your truth.

Find a practitioner of Kinesiology or Dowsing, and/or learn these techniques yourself for testing purposes.

Receive Loving Human Touch, and learn Self Massage and Progressive Relaxation.

Connect with the Divine, whatever that may be for you.

Consider your Lineage, Family History and Life Style.

Learn how to Google as a way of informing yourself!

Check List for Cancer Diagnosis

I recommend reading the following books to begin your Journey – or have someone else read them for you and share with you the information, so you can make some choices about your treatment. Please ask for the latest edition. There is no need to panic, or rush into anything, in most cases. Take time to make decisions, and ask questions so as to be informed. Write the answers, or better still, have someone do that for you. Keep a special book for this purpose – possibly an indexed book – for taking notes on your information.

Cancer Explained by Professor Fred Stephens and Richard Fox

How to Prevent and Treat Cancer with Natural Medicine by Dr. Michael Murray, Dr. Tim Birdsall, Dr. Joseph E. Pizzorno and Dr. Paul Reilly

An Alternative Medicine Definitive Guide to Cancer by Burton Goldberg

The Acid Alkaline Diet for Optimal Health by Christopher Vasey N.D.

Cancer Free by Bill Henderson

Cancer Recovery Guide: 15 Alternative and Complementary Strategies for Restoring Health by Jonathan Chamberlain

The Choice: The Programme by Bernadette Bohan

Cancer: Step Outside the Box by Ty M. Bolinger

Foods To Fight Cancer by Professor Richard Beliveau and Dr. Denis Gingras

Cancer: Cause and Cure by Percy Weston

The Secret by Rhonda Byrne

Find one person who has the time, energy and willingness to be your Buddy through this time, professional or otherwise. This person will do what needs to be done, order what needs to be ordered, and get you as much support as possible. She, or he, will know how to delegate and organize offers of help, and when to say no. All of your energy and time will go toward your healing, and learning how to receive that. Each person and situation is unique, and you must explore what is right for you on a daily basis.

Check the benefits from your health insurance.

If counselling services of any kind are covered by your insurance policy do consider availing of this. If you are not covered and can afford it please find a psychotherapist of your choosing to support you. Ask for a referral.

Local cancer societies often offer counselling and useful advice. Our minds, emotions and subconscious influence our lives more than is realized. Energy follows thought, and so it is of the utmost importance to keep a positive attitude. This can be difficult in the case of a cancer diagnosis, and so a Buddy, Counsellor and/or Coach are invaluable allies in this very challenging time.

Our state of mind can make the difference between life and death.

Check out the following websites...

Google your national or local cancer website and call to talk to someone.

www.canceractive.com a charity website for good guidelines on all aspects of cancer therapy.

www.cancertutor.com for access to much information on treatment guidelines for cancer.

www.cancerfightingstrategies.com for more information given clearly and comprehensively.

www.cancertruth.com for information on exploring the truth about cancer cause and cure.

www.cancerx.org for the most knowledge on healing cancer with digestive enzymes. They have a formula which they will give you when you call.

www.huldaclark.org for effective ways to clear parasites as well as other helpful information to heal cancer.

If you wish to opt for an alternative route, and can afford it, choose a cancer clinic and go and stay there, or nearby. There are some listed in the book Cancer Free by Bill Hendersen, and Cancer: Step Outside the Box by Ty M Bolinger, and on the web. Some will use Conventional and Alternative Medicine, while others will just use Alternative. The best ones will give you a choice, or assess you and help you to make your decisions.

One of the most important things you can do is to take care of your immune system. Some possible ways are with supplements such as ProBiotics, Beta-Glucans, Green Powders, Raw Juices and Enzymes, Echinacea, Chinese Herbs, Colloidal Trace Minerals and other supplements, as well as laughter and life style changes. Each person is unique, and regardless of what might be generally recommended, it is advisable to find a practitioner who will test you for your needs. Some people can learn to do this for themselves very successfully and quickly with dowsing or kinesiology, and this can be used on a daily basis, in conjunction with your practitioner. The choice is yours, but if more stress is caused by this it is not a good idea. Doing it all by yourself is not a wise choice for most people, though some may want that total self focus, which definitely has its benefits, as long as you have some kind of plan to follow.

Watching funny movies has been shown to improve your immune system

If you are following a conventional medical path you will need to consult with them if you intend to take supplements in case of contraindications.

Ways to change as soon as possible…

There are certain foods that feed cancer, so it is wise to stop eating them. They are as follows…

Sugar, all processed foods, all foods not grown organically (having too much phosphate and an imbalance of minerals) alcohol, dairy products (which produce mucus relished by cancer cells) caffeine, tap water, and most meat until you are healed, and then you can choose after this. If Metastases is present extra protein is needed. See **www.cancerx.org**

The major trick is to keep your system alkaline with alkaline forming foods, alkalising water and stress reduction. Cancer or any disease does not live in an alkaline body. Learn about this process in the book Acid and Alkaline by Herman Aihara or google acid alkaline diet simplified.

Find some spiritual focus – explore, explore, and follow your heart.

Bless your food and everything else. It can become a positive mantra.

Breathe…breathe…breathe…breathing will teach you.

Exercise…exercise…exercise…

Exercise will detox you, amongst many other things. Find your own comfort zone.

May your Soul benefit enormously from this adventure called Cancer.

May you remember that you are made up of many different parts, most of which are very healthy and happy.

May you know that you are Love and Loved – and that "the only constant is change!"

Conclusion

Writing this book has not been an easy task for me, mostly because my energy has been given to what I needed to do to balance my Soul, imbalance of which has caused my disease. I am not quite there yet, but almost………I am a stubborn creature. It has served me well, as well as causing me challenges. I understand it quite well now and know that that part of me needs constant coaching and accountability.

I have undertaken to share my experience of healing from cancer because the teacher in me is somewhat compulsive. If I find something that I think is helpful, and brings more truth to this world I want to talk or write about it. Many of us feel the same, and I am grateful to all those who have shared their findings on cancer, from all walks of life.

Cancer does not discriminate regarding gender, age, race, religion or education. It is ultimately an opportunity to face oneself and to know love, peace and truth, inside and out, however one does the journey. It is also an opportunity to explore one's creativity and how that wants to express itself out into the world. This is something we have always known but parts have been held back. We have **resisted** our next steps, for whatever reason, from fear, greed or laziness. Then comes the **resentment** towards ourselves (perhaps projected onto others), the **conflict** and the **despair**. These repressed feelings have a lot to answer for, so it serves us well to allow them a voice.

At this time in history energy has speeded up, so we can take advantage of this to hasten our own healing. The bottom line is finding the happiness that is our birthright moment to moment.

May all Beings be Happy, as the Buddha said.

Balancing my Soul required me to act on what I knew was needed for this goal. I needed to live alone, for however long, which necessitated leaving my partner and trailmate of nine years and thirty three years living in America. My native Ireland called. The Earth herself called me, as she does all of us, when we listen. I surrendered with much grief, and also joy. They can live side by side.

My family called, and I needed and wanted them also. It has been very challenging, with many awarenesses and much gratitude. I am preparing for the next lap of the journey, eager to do my part in raising the vibration of this beautiful Planet Earth in the ways that I know how, and using the gifts that I have been given. As I learn how to access more of my own gifts and truth I am able to help others access theirs. This makes me very happy.

I have been, and am, journeying back to Source with a lot of help and support from many. Each encounter brings a gift, however it may appear – each a reflection for me – an opportunity to resist projection and blame, to embrace love and compassion for myself as well as others, to see myself and to change in whatever way is beneficial to bring me to wholeness. Most of all, with each encounter is the opportunity for joy. Each person vibrating joy ripples it out to everyone, beyond loss, beyond recession, beyond anger and beyond despair, so let us find it with each other as we find it in ourselves.

Each of us has a unique calling in the grand scheme of things, however small it may look. Little things mean a lot and can often be life saving, individually, collectively and globally.

"God Bless" as we say many times a day here in Ireland - one of the wonderful things about returning home. I am blessed often by this phrase on the phone, in the shops and saying goodbye and now want to pass it on to you also.

Heather

Some Suggestions for Using These Pages

• Appointments • Important Phone Numbers • Affirmations • Daily Practice
• Medications/Supplements • Exercise • Diet • Journaling • Books
• Goals/Intentions • CDs & DVDs • Websites

Notes

Notes

Notes

Notes

Notes

Notes

Notes

Notes

Notes

Notes

Notes

Notes